The oxygen Diet Solution

YOUR ULTIMATE 28-DAY SHAPE-UP PLAN

Dr. Susan Kleiner

RD, FACN, CNS, FISSN

with the editors of *Oxygen* magazine

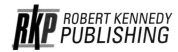

ROBERT KENNEDY PUBLISHING

Published by Robert Kennedy Publishing
400 Matheson Blvd. West
Mississauga, ON
L5R 3M1 Canada
Visit us at www.rkpubs.com
and www.oxygenmag.com

Kleiner, Susan M.
   The Oxygen diet solution : your ultimate
28-day shape-up plan / Susan Kleiner ; with the
editors of Oxygen magazine.

Includes index.
ISBN 978-1-55210-122-3

   1. Reducing diets--Recipes. 2. Weight loss.
3. Physical fitness. I. Title.

RM222.2.K571 2012   613.2'5
C2012-906336-3

10 9 8 7 6 5 4 3 2 1

Distributed in Canada by
NBN (National Book Network)
67 Mowat Avenue, Suite 241
Toronto, ON
M6K 3E3

Distributed in USA by
NBN (National Book Network)
15200 NBN Way
Blue Ridge Summit, PA
17214

Printed in Canada

Robert Kennedy Publishing
BOOK DEPARTMENT

MANAGING DIRECTOR
Wendy Morley

SENIOR EDITOR
Amy Land

EDITOR, ONLINE AND PRINT
Meredith Barrett

ASSOCIATE EDITOR
Rachel Corradetti

ONLINE EDITOR
Kiersten Corradetti

EDITORIAL ASSISTANT
Brittany Seki

ART DIRECTOR
Gabriella Caruso Marques

INTERIM ART DIRECTOR
Jessica Hearn

SENIOR DESIGNER
Brian Ross

PROP/WARDROBE STYLIST
Kelsey-Lynn Corradetti

SENIOR WEB DESIGNER
Christopher Barnes

EXECUTIVE ASSISTANT
Jeannie Mahoney

INDEXING
James De Medeiros

WITH:
Diane Hart, Editor in Chief, Oxygen Special Issues & Digital Content
Stacy Rinella, Editor in Chief, Oxygen Magazine
Alaina Chapman, Designer, Oxygen Magazine
Paul Buceta, Oxygen's Chief Photographer

WRITTEN BY:
Susan Kleiner, Wendy Morley, Amy Land,
Meredith Barrett and Brittany Seki

IMPORTANT

The information in this book reflects the author's
experiences and opinions and is not intended to
replace medical advice.

Before beginning this or any nutritional or exercise
regimen, consult your physician to be sure it is
appropriate for you. Ask for a physical stress test.

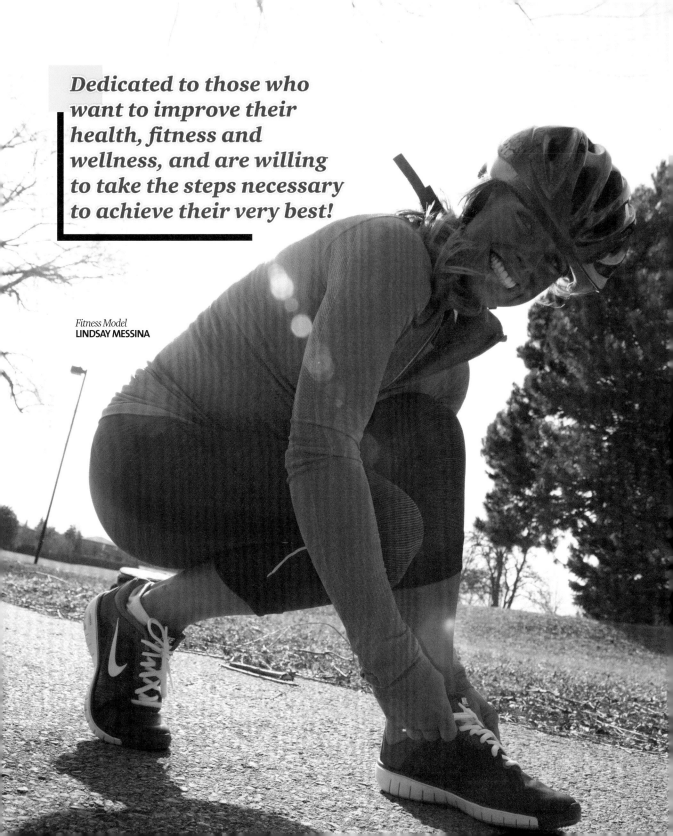

Dedicated to those who want to improve their health, fitness and wellness, and are willing to take the steps necessary to achieve their very best!

Fitness Model
LINDSAY MESSINA

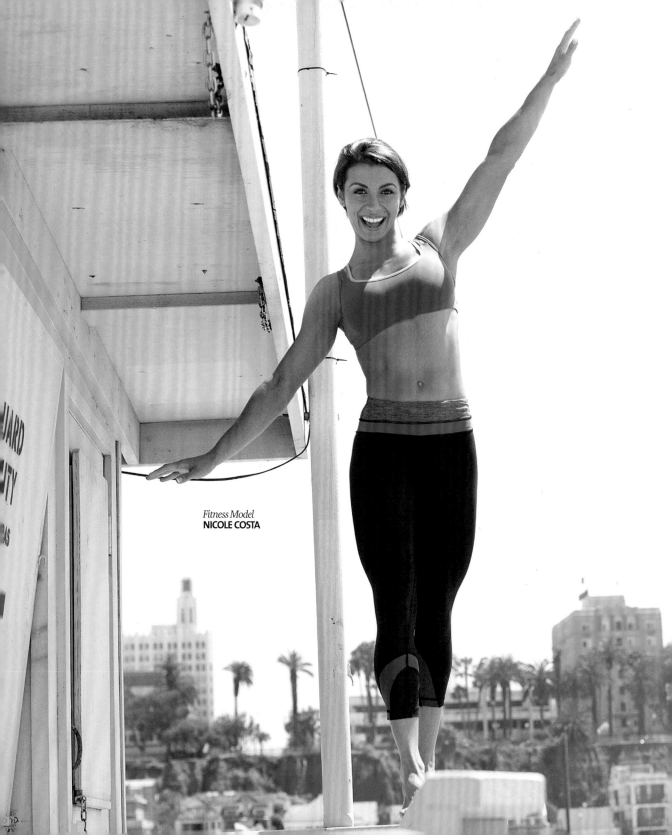

Fitness Model
NICOLE COSTA

> **If you have a passion for life and all it offers, does the quest for self-improvement ever stop?**
> — ROBERT KENNEDY, *OXYGEN* FOUNDER

TABLE OF CONTENTS

INTRODUCTION

On any given day at *Oxygen* headquarters there is no shortage of clean foods. Editors and artists stock up the lunchroom with plenty of meals and snacks to get them through the workday. Mornings consist of hard-boiled eggs or egg whites, oatmeal, a variety of nut butters and anti-oxidant-loaded fruits such as blueberries, raspberries and blackberries. Fast forward to lunch hour. The most common meal is salad. Boring? No way! Mixed greens with plenty of colorful, nutrient-loaded veggies such as tomatoes and bell peppers topped with chickpeas and protein, usually tuna or chicken. Toss an avocado into the mix for a dose of healthy fats, half a whole-wheat pita or sweet potato on the side, and you've got a clean lunch to keep you full until snack time two to three hours later.

When we all go home at night, our meals look something like this: ground turkey lettuce wraps, asparagus and turkey muffins, black bean burgers, and homemade salsa with salmon. Chances are we already have our clean meals planned (and possibly prepped) way in advance, so it's just a matter of cooking. No last-minute runs to the grocery store. Any seasoned clean eater knows planning and prep work is more than half the battle.

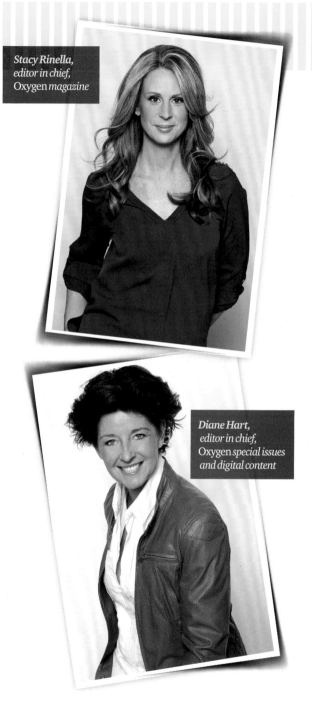

Stacy Rinella,
editor in chief,
Oxygen *magazine*

Diane Hart,
editor in chief,
Oxygen *special issues*
and digital content

A stellar diet is crucial to get and keep the body you've always wanted. But any *Oxygen* gal knows fitness plays a key role as well. We're in the gym four or five days a week, breaking it down into resistance training and cardio sessions. Some of us even manage to add Pilates and yoga classes to our weekly regimens. Sure we look good, but bonus, this lifestyle has us feeling great too.

While we now have it down to a fine science, we weren't born with this knowledge. Before *Oxygen* magazine came into our lives, many of us were eating the wrong foods at the wrong times. Not to mention what we were or were *not* doing in the gym. But luckily, thanks to the resources at our disposal, we've nailed it. And we're happy to share this knowledge with you!

In this book you will find guidance, no matter what your fitness and nutrition goals may be. Need to lose 30 lbs? Check. Want to improve your health through eating well? Check, check. And if you happen to be in great shape and just looking for ways to maintain and fine tune, we've got that too! We went to the best in the fitness biz – *Oxygen*'s cover and workout models – to get their nutrition, fitness and health tips. With bods like theirs they must be doing something right!

Boost immunity, build muscle, increase your energy, beat stress, plus you'll love all the recipes, workouts and advice to get you on the right path and help you stay there! You'll love this book!

Getting Started

Your Total Transformation Solution

There's a common misconception that a "diet" has to be some drastic and unpleasant change in your eating habits that results in weight loss while you're "on" it. Often the person going on a diet expects to give up or almost give up one food group or another, possibly take some sort of magic pill, potion, drink or special food, and probably go very, very hungry.

If you're like most people, you've tried one, two or maybe even 20 of these types of diets before. It's worth stating here that normally people who try one of these diets soon find themselves trying another (and another, and so on …) because they are a temporary solution to a permanent problem. In fact, a deprivation-type diet is your quickest route to a lowered metabolism. Not only that, but usually most of the weight you lose, at least at the outset, is water weight. Lucky for all of us, the science of fat burning has shown that starvation is not the way to go.

Permanent Weight Loss and Good Health

If you've ever read an issue of *Oxygen* magazine, you'll know we promote a diet that provides fat loss, yes, but also one that provides the nutrients that keep your body healthy, vibrant and functioning at its best. We know that lifelong fat loss and optimal health is the way to go, not short-term fat and water loss, and then rebounding with fat gain, reduced metabolism and guilt. It's not at all uncommon for people following *Oxygen*'s eating plans to find that they eat more while losing weight than they did while they were gaining weight. It's simply a matter of choosing the right foods and eating them at specified times (including NOT skipping meals!).

Timing and combining of nutrients was first shown to be profoundly important in my area of specialty, sports nutrition. It became clear that eating protein and carbohydrates separately had a different effect on the body when compared to eating protein and carbs together. Carbohydrates are anabolic, meaning they help you store muscle fuel and build tissues and other important elements of the body: enzymes, immune factors and so on. Proteins are not only the building blocks for all of these compounds, but they also catalyze these reactions, meaning they can speed up the whole process – like putting your finger directly on the hot button versus cranking a wheel.

Proteins and carbohydrates also work together in your brain to build serotonin levels, supporting your mood, mental focus and sense of energy. By adding high-performance fats into the mix every time you eat (except before and after exercise), you not only slow down the pace of digestion to keep your blood sugar levels balanced and even, you bathe your brain, central nervous system and entire body with important anti-inflammatory compounds that promote tissue recovery and repair for better health and performance. Healthy fats also help elevate your mood and enhance your memory.

Every meal and snack of each diet in this book is designed with nutrient timing and combining in mind. You will also get the micronutrients, phytochemicals, fiber and food factors that promote health and prevent disease. So even though the goal of your diet may be weight loss, your health, along with physical and mental performance, is never sidelined. No one knows how to alter your body composition and body weight like a seasoned high-performance nutritionist. That is why *The Oxygen Diet Solution* is different – and that is why it works as no other diet can. Because your ultimate goal is not just weight loss but also how you feel and perform, I've designed *The Oxygen Diet Solution* so that you can have it all.

Dr. Susan Kleiner, RD, FACN, CNS, FISSN

Where to begin? Decide which of the following profiles best matches your current needs and then flip to the corresponding section, where your solution awaits!

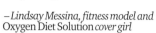

YOUR GOAL | YOUR DIET

"I've got an upcoming event that I need to look super-hot for – fast!"	**Quick Fat-Loss Diet,** p. 40
"I have more than 15 pounds to lose."	**The Basic *Oxygen* Diet,** p. 18
"I want to build sexy toned muscles."	**Muscle-Building Diet,** p. 90
"I want to work out, but I barely have the energy to make it through the day."	**Super-Energy Diet,** p. 56
"I can't miss another day of work! Why do I keep getting sick?"	**Power-Immunity Diet,** p. 72
"I've lost the weight and want to start seeing some definition."	**Muscle-Building Diet,** p. 90
"Yippee! I've lost the weight!! Now I need to keep it off!"	**The Basic *Oxygen* Diet,** p. 18

NOTE: For vegan and gluten-free substitutions, see p. 278.

Fitting it All In

THE *OXYGEN* STAFF SHARE THEIR SECRETS TO SUCCESS!

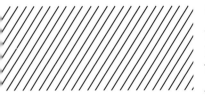

"Don't say you don't have enough time. You have exactly the same number of hours per day that were given to Helen Keller, Pasteur, Michelangelo, Mother Teresa, Leonardo da Vinci, Thomas Jefferson, and Albert Einstein."

– *H. Jackson Brown Jr., author of* Life's Little Instruction Book

As you are about to embark on the diet of your choice, you might be apprehensive about how on earth you're going to manage five or six workouts each week, plus preparing all this new food, on top of working full time, commuting, bringing the kids to soccer and dance, helping them with homework, and having a fulfilling relationship with your partner. It's easy to just skip the workout and grab some fast food when life is this busy, but you don't want to make excuses – you want to succeed! And you *can* succeed at doing all this, and more. The key is to plan, to be organized and most importantly, to be committed.

Changing your routine can take some time and effort, but with these tips from the super-savvy *Oxygen* team, you'll be able to stay on track until these healthy habits eventually become second nature to you. As late *Oxygen* founder Robert Kennedy said, "Failure is not an option!"

1 / Plan your weekly meals in advance.

Our food plans make this much easier for you, but you may have to switch some meals around or you may have to plan a different meal for yourself than for your family (though it's best to keep that to a minimum). Don't wait until the last minute to figure out your meals or you will be that much more likely to go off your diet.

"Planning is paramount. On Sunday, take a look at your weekly schedule and figure out when, what and how you'll train. Then figure out what you'll need for breakfast, lunch, dinner and snacking, and make food you can freeze and take with you for the rest of the week."

– Dave Bowden, managing editor

2 / Pack your lunch and snacks.

This takes just a few minutes each evening but helps to ensure your success. If you know you have a meal waiting for you, you are far less likely to succumb to temptation.

"When it comes to my lunches, on Sundays I make one huge salad that will last me for the whole workweek. I take a little bit out every day and add a protein and homemade dressing."

– Natalie Amaral, senior designer

3 / Freeze!

Frozen fruits and vegetables are just as nutritious as fresh, and they can be a real time-saver. Also, cooking larger batches and freezing them in smaller portions is a great idea. Take your evening meal out in the morning to thaw – there's nothing better than coming home to a dinner that's already made!

"Making planned leftovers is a great way to ensure that you always have clean meals on hand."

– Tosca Reno, Oxygen columnist, author, motivational speaker and fitness model

4 / Always have good choices on hand.

Make extra chicken breasts, salad and anything else you will be eating a lot of. This is a huge time-saver, and when you find yourself getting home late you'll be very happy you don't have to cook!

"I always make sure that with every meal and snack I have some kind of protein to keep me full. I always eat breakfast no matter what, and I always keep healthy snacks at my desk so I don't let myself go hungry."

– Erin Lutz, assistant art director

5 / Schedule your workouts.

Don't let anything get in the way. There are 168 hours in each week; you can take a mere six of those hours to ensure your success in weight loss and health.

"Create a routine! Hitting the gym at the same time every day can make it easier to incorporate into your busy schedule – treat it like an appointment you can't miss!"

– Savithri Sastri, online editor

6 / Exercise during your lunch hour.

If you work at a business that allows you to eat at your desk, lunch hour is a great time to train. Not only are you making the best use of your valuable time, a midday workout will give you tons more energy to get through the afternoon. Yes, really!

"Working at Oxygen makes it fairly easy to stay on track. An in-office gym, shower facilities and lunchtime running groups all help make working out convenient – and convenience is key for me!"

– Alaina Chapman, designer

7 / Be mindful.

Half an hour of focused attention is better than three hours of semi-attention. When you are working out, be in the workout. Feel your body moving. Appreciate it. When you are with your family, be truly with them. A little goes a much longer way when that little is filled with quality.

"I've been on countless food sets for Oxygen magazine and with each experience comes more knowledge and understanding of eating clean and the positive effect it can have on your life."

– Stacy Jarvis, art director

8 / Ditch the guilt.

Plenty of women feel guilty for looking after themselves, but ask yourself this: Do those you love want you to be around for a long time? Of course they do! Looking after yourself is a gift to you and also a gift to them. Be sure to remind yourself of this when you start to feel guilty.

"Flip your to-do list so that you are on top all the time. I know it seems selfish, but you can't take care of others unless you take care of yourself first.

– Marta Ustyanich, copy editor

9 / Get enough sleep.

Sure, fitting sleep in along with everything else takes some work, but getting enough sleep will make everything else run much more smoothly. Those who don't get enough sleep are more likely to gain weight and less likely to stick to their diet and exercise plans. Plus, sleeping enough makes you look and feel better – they don't call it "beauty sleep" for nothing!

"A lack of sleep not only drains my energy, but makes it hard to concentrate. That's when my workouts suffer and I give in to cravings for comfort foods. Being well-rested is key for staying focused on my goals."

– Kirstyn Brown, nutrition editor

10 / Use your screen time wisely.

It's amazing how easily the TV, computer, smartphone and tablet can suck you in. We've all had times when we've gone to the computer to check our email and end up wasting a couple of hours watching YouTube videos. When you do browse, make sure you are checking out sites that will help you on your way to your best body (Hint: Oxygenmag.com)!

"I follow a lot of fitness models and fitness-related companies on Facebook, so I'm flooded with inspiration daily. Kim Lyons and Kim Dolan Leto are two of my personal faves."

– Ashley Souter, designer

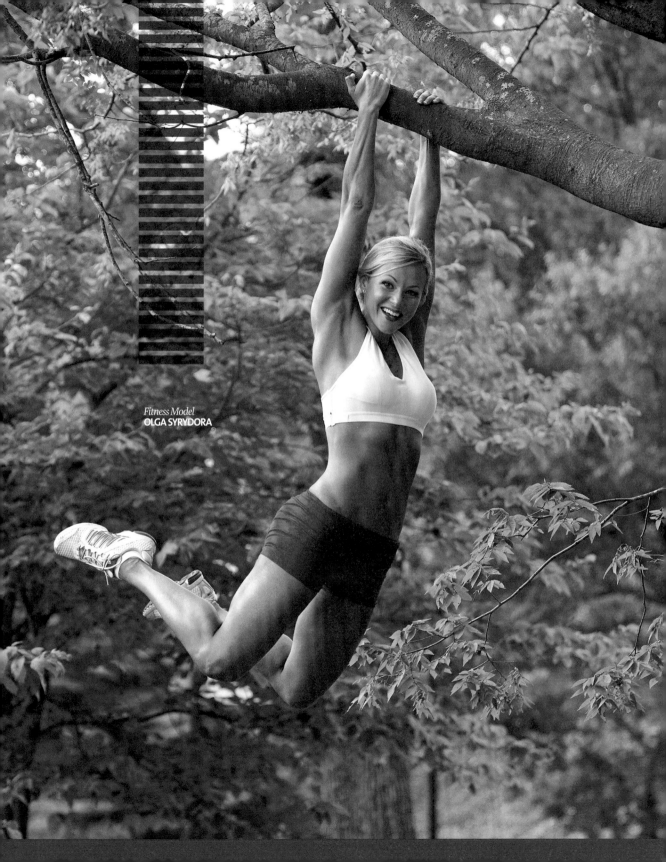

Fitness Model
OLGA SYRYDORA

PART I

THE DIETS

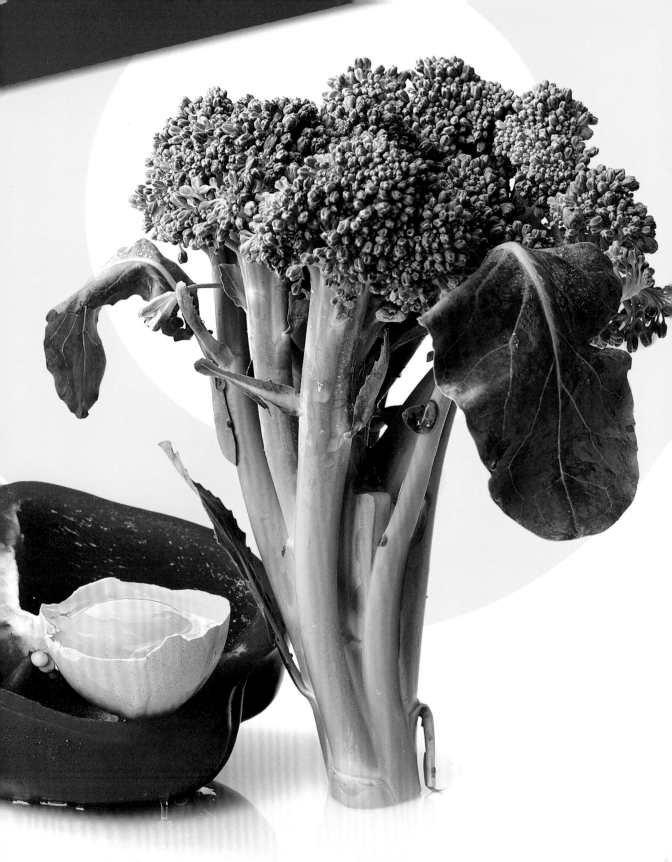

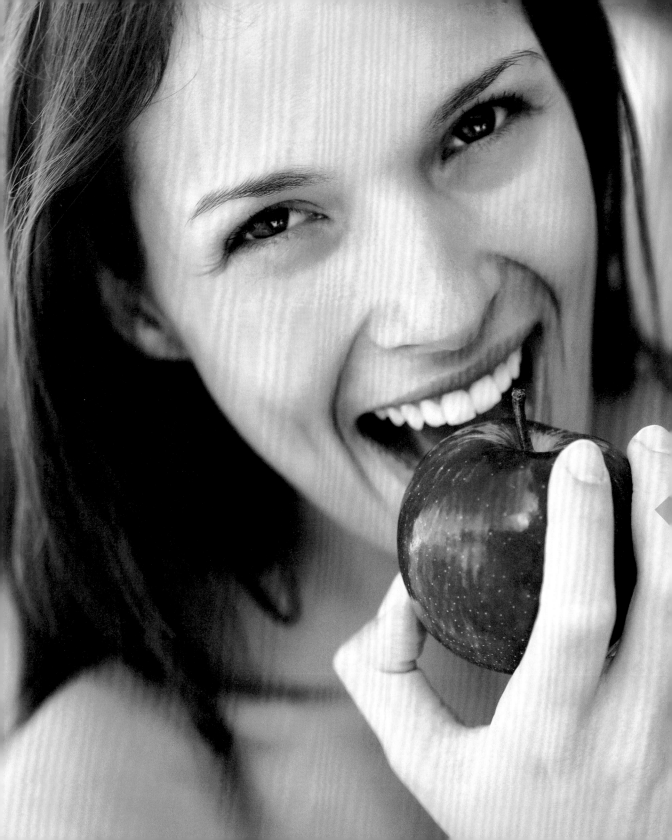

The Basic Oxygen Diet

To drop more than 10 pounds and for long-term weight maintenance

If you have more than 10 pounds to lose, or if you've lost all your excess weight (congratulations!) and are now looking to maintain, then The Basic Diet is the one for you. Our Basic *Oxygen* Diet gives you exactly what you need for steady weight loss, and with a few small adjustments will help you keep that weight off for the rest of your life. Yes, you will finally be able to throw out your "fat" clothes for good!

Our Basic *Oxygen* Diet offers enough calories to fuel the five or six workouts you'll do each week as part of this program. It will help you have the energy to do those workouts. You'll get plenty of food, so you won't feel hungry. And you'll be providing your body with all the nutrients – macro and micro – it needs to thrive.

But don't feel that you are limited to the Basic *Oxygen* Diet. The diets in this book will all help you achieve fat loss and good health, so feel free to try the others. If you have been losing weight steadily for a few weeks or more and find that you've plateaued, do the Quick Fat-Loss Diet for a couple of weeks and you should break through that pound barrier. Or maybe you've lost quite a bit of weight and want to start seeing some definition; then the Muscle-Building Diet is exactly what you need (with some muscle-building exercise, of course!).

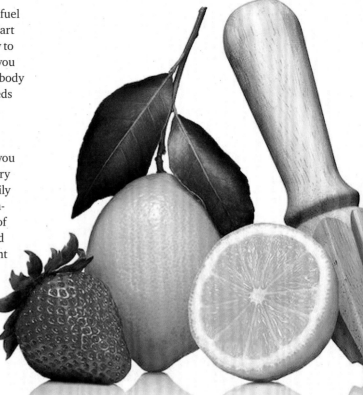

If I'm maintaining my weight, why am I on a diet?

Does it surprise you that the same diet is used for losing weight as for maintenance? You might be surprised because of your preconceived idea about what the word "diet" means. Diet just means eating plan, period. Whatever you eat on a regular basis is your diet.

In the case of people who need to lose weight, their diet has been providing them with excessive calories and probably unhealthy choices. In the case of people who are lean and fit, their diets provide adequate calories for their daily activities. Some people are underweight, and their diets do not provide enough calories. But all this is just talking about body size and calories. While size is relevant, being healthy and feeling good is about much more than that! And with the diets in this book, you will achieve all these goals!

Your Basic *Oxygen* Diet Meal Plan

Are you ready? Here is your two-week Basic Diet. Follow it twice for the 28-day plan, or you can continue to follow it indefinitely for long-term weight loss and weight maintenance. You don't have to follow every day as set out here – you can swap any meal for the same meal on another day. In other words, you can choose any lunch to eat as your lunch, but you cannot choose a dinner option as your lunch. This diet is 45.5 percent carbs, 30 percent fats and 24.5 percent protein.

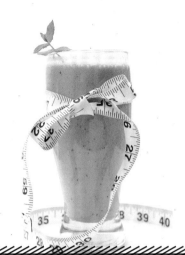

Snack Time!

In addition to the three meals per day listed in The Basic *Oxygen* Diet meal plan, you can have two daily snacks. These can be around exercise (one before and one after) or if you are not working out then one in the morning and one in the afternoon.

Optimally you will place the pre- and postworkout snacks exactly before and after you exercise, whenever that is during the day. However, if you exercise immediately after a meal or within 30 minutes of your next meal, move the pre- and/or postworkout snacks to another time during the day when a snack will break up a period of longer than three hours between meals.

SNACK 1
- 1 cup plain low-fat yogurt (not Greek)
- ½ cup fresh berries, halved
- ⅛ ounce (about 1 tbsp) slivered or sliced almonds

SNACK 2
Smoothie – blend together:
- 1 cup nonfat milk
- ½ fresh banana (frozen is best)
- ½ cup frozen berries
- ½ scoop (10 grams) whey protein isolate (look for one with no additives)

SNACK 3
- One serving of Almond Butter Whey Cookies (p. 270)

SWEET TREATS
Once per week, you can treat yourself with **one serving** of only one of these snacks:

Preworkout
- Mini Chocolate Soufflés (p. 269)

Postworkout
- Peppermint Protein Ice Cream (p. 273)
- Chocolate Power Pudding (p. 274)

For more tips on treats, see p. 183.

THE BASIC *OXYGEN* DIET MEAL PLAN

BEFORE YOU BEGIN:

Follow this meal plan twice for the 28-day plan.

If the variety of the plan has you feeling overwhelmed, you can choose a few of your favorites and then repeat them. You can swap one breakfast for another, or one lunch for another, or one dinner for another. But don't swap dinner for lunch, or breakfast for dinner and so on.

If absolutely necessary, you can also switch the order of meals within one day, but ideally you should not.

* You will be having the Simple Dressing on an almost daily basis. For recipe, see p. 24.

** This fish dish can be substituted with the Grilled Raspberry Salmon on p. 266.

DAY 1

BREAKFAST
Omelette: In a nonstick pan, cook 1 egg + 1 tbsp chopped onions or scallions + 2 tbsp diced tomato; 1 slice whole-grain toast; ½ cup orange juice; 2 cups water; coffee/tea

LUNCH
Large salad: 2 cups mixed greens + ½ cup sliced cucumber + ¼ cup sliced mushrooms + ¼ cup diced red pepper + ⅓ cup diced avocado + 2 oz grilled chicken, sliced + Simple Dressing*; 4–6 (½ oz) low-fat whole wheat crackers or crispbreads; 1 apple; 2 cups water; tea/other non-caloric beverage

DINNER
Grilled fish**: 3 oz grilled fish of your choice, seasoned with 1 tsp EVOO (extra-virgin olive oil) + ½ tbsp lemon juice, sea salt, pepper; 12 asparagus spears grilled with 1 tsp EVOO + crushed garlic; **Large salad:** 1 cup mixed greens + 1 cup raw spinach + ½ cup mung bean sprouts + 3 cherry tomatoes + 1 tbsp chopped Italian parsley + 1 tbsp toasted sliced almonds + Simple Dressing*; ⅓ cup cooked quinoa; 2 cups water; tea/other non-caloric beverage

DAY 2

BREAKFAST
Egg tortilla: In a nonstick pan, lightly sauté 1 tbsp minced shallots + 2 tbsp shredded zucchini + 1 tbsp chopped red pepper + 1 egg, slightly beaten. Add egg mixture and 2 tbsp salsa to a 6-inch whole wheat tortilla; ½ cup pineapple juice; 2 cups water; coffee/tea

LUNCH
Chicken veggie stir-fry (see tip, p. 24): Sauté 2 oz chicken breast strips + 3 cups sliced mixed vegetables + 1½ tsp peanut oil + 2 tsp minced garlic + ½ tsp sesame seeds + 1 tbsp low-sodium soy sauce (add at end of cooking); ⅔ cup brown rice; 1 orange; 2 cups water; tea/other non-caloric beverage

DINNER
Scallops (or other seafood) with beets and greens: Lightly sauté 3 oz sea scallops + 1½ tsp olive oil + ½ tbsp minced garlic; steam 2 cups Swiss chard + 1 cup cubed golden or red beets + toss with ½ tsp olive oil and herbs; ⅓ cup polenta; **Small salad:** 1 cup mixed greens + sliced radishes + 1 tbsp chopped parsley + 1 small tomato, sliced + Simple Dressing*; 2 cups water; tea/other non-caloric beverage

DAY 3

BREAKFAST
Sunshine Breakfast Shake (p. 209); 2 cups water; coffee/tea

LUNCH
Large tuna salad: 2 cups mixed greens + ½ cup steamed green string beans + 3 red onion rings + 3 cherry tomatoes + 2 oz fresh grilled or canned tuna + Simple Dressing*; 4–6 (½ oz) low-fat whole wheat crackers or crispbreads; 1 cup mixed berries; 2 cups water; tea/other non-caloric beverage

DINNER
Halibut stir-fry (see tip, p. 24): Sauté raw garlic + ½ cup mushrooms + 2 tbsp onions + 1 stalk chopped celery + 1 cup snow peas + 3 oz sliced halibut filet seasoned with low-sodium soy sauce, ginger and 1 tsp canola oil in nonstick wok or pan; ⅓ cup cooked quinoa; **Large salad:** 1 cup shredded red and green cabbage + 1 cup shredded Bok Choy + Simple Dressing*; 2 cups water; Tea/other non-caloric beverage

DAY 4

BREAKFAST
½ cup cottage cheese mixed with 2 tbsp shredded carrot + 2 tbsp chopped cucumber + 2 tbsp shredded broccoli stalk or celery + 1 tbsp chopped parsley, salt and pepper to taste; 1 slice whole-grain toast; ½ cup pineapple juice; 2 cups water; coffee/tea

LUNCH
EAT OUT! Vietnamese restaurant: Order sweet and sour fish stew + 2 fresh vegetable salad rolls; fresh fruit cup; 2 cups water; tea/other non-caloric beverage

DINNER
Lamb chops and greens: 3 oz grilled lamb chops + 1 cup roasted Brussels sprouts (tossed in ½ tsp EVOO); 1 cup winter squash or ½ cup yam; Large salad: 2 cups mixed greens + ½ cup sliced cucumber + ¼ cup sliced mushrooms + ¼ cup diced red pepper + 1 tbsp diced avocado + Simple Dressing*; 2 cups water; tea/other non-caloric beverage

DAY 5

BREAKFAST
Egg lettuce rolls: 2–3 large iceberg lettuce leaves + 1 hard-boiled egg, diced + 1 tbsp shredded carrot + 1 tbsp diced celery, mixed with 1 tsp reduced-fat mayonnaise + ½ tsp yellow mustard. Place ½ egg mixture into lettuce cup and roll up; ½ fresh grapefruit; 2 cups water; coffee/tea

LUNCH
Chicken sandwich: 2 oz sliced grilled chicken breast or deli chicken + lettuce leaves and tomato slices + 3 avocado slices + mustard on 2 slices whole-grain bread; Mixed greens salad + Simple Dressing*; apple; 2 cups water; tea/other non-caloric beverage

DINNER
Steak with olive tapenade and cucumber: 3 oz grilled tenderloin + ½ cup sautéed mushrooms and onions, 1½ cups chard + 1 tsp EVOO and garlic; 1 tbsp olive tapenade + ½ cup sliced cucumber (spread tapenade on cucumber slices); 1 cup winter squash or ½ cup yam; Large salad: 1 ½ cups mixed greens + 6 sliced radishes + 1 tbsp fresh chopped parsley + 1 small tomato, sliced + Simple Dressing*; 2 cups water; tea/other non-caloric beverage

DAY 6

BREAKFAST
1 egg prepared any way; 1 slice whole-grain toast topped with 1–2 tbsp plain yogurt, sliced tomato and cucumber; ½ fresh grapefruit; 2 cups water; coffee/tea

LUNCH
Tuna salad sandwich: 2 oz tuna + 1 dill pickle, finely chopped + ¼ tsp minced ginger + ¼ tsp curry powder + 1 tsp reduced-fat mayonnaise + lettuce leaves on 2 slices whole-grain bread; sliced mixed vegetables on the side; 1 cup cubed melon; 2 cups water; tea/other non-caloric beverage

DINNER
Chicken Sautéed with Leeks & Arugula (p. 246); Large salad: 2 cups mixed greens + ½ cup steamed green string beans + 3 red onion slices + 3 cherry tomatoes + Simple Dressing*; 2 cups water; tea/other non-caloric beverage

DAY 7

BREAKFAST
Egg foo young omelette: In a nonstick pan, cook 1 egg + 2 tbsp chopped scallions + ¼ cup mung bean sprouts + ¼ cup sliced mushrooms + ⅓ cup cooked brown rice + ½ tsp low-sodium soy sauce; ½ cup orange juice; 2 cups water; coffee/tea

LUNCH
Turkey salad: 2 oz sliced turkey breast + 2 cups mixed greens + 1 stalk chopped celery + ½ cup broccoli florets + 1 tbsp toasted sunflower seeds + Simple Dressing*; 4–6 (½ oz) low-fat whole wheat crackers or crispbreads; 1 orange; 2 cups water; tea/other non-caloric beverage

DINNER
Sirloin burger with layered salad: 3 oz broiled sirloin burger + lettuce, tomato, onion, mustard and 2 tsp ketchup on 1 whole-grain slider bun; 12 asparagus spears tossed with minced garlic and grilled; Layer together 1 medium tomato, sliced + fresh basil leaves + drizzle with ½ tsp EVOO + 1 tsp balsamic vinegar; 2 cups water; tea/other non-caloric beverage

THE BASIC *OXYGEN* DIET MEAL PLAN

SIMPLE DRESSING

You will be eating a large salad almost every day topped with this fat-blasting vinaigrette mix.

1 tbsp extra virgin olive oil

2 tsp red wine vinegar

Sea salt and pepper, to taste

Mix all ingredients in a small bowl or mason jar. Pour over salad. Makes 1 serving. You can make a larger batch and measure out one 1½-tbsp serving per salad.

*Nutrients per serving:
Calories: 126, Total Fat: 14 g,
Saturated fat: 2 g, Trans Fat: 0 g,
Cholesterol: 0 mg, Sodium: 8.5 mg,
Total Carbohydrates: 0 g,
Dietary Fiber: 0 g, Sugars: 0 g,
Protein: 0 g, Iron: 0 mg*

STIR-FRY TIP

When a stir-fry recipe calls for mixed vegetables, feel free to use any combination of the following abs-firming picks: broccoli, onions, carrots, zucchini, red pepper, red cabbage, mushrooms, snow peas, water chestnuts and bean sprouts.

DAY 8

BREAKFAST
Egg tortilla: In a nonstick pan, lightly sauté 1 tbsp minced shallots + 2 tbsp shredded zucchini + 1 tbsp chopped red pepper + 1 egg, slightly beaten; Add egg mixture and 2 tbsp salsa to a 6-inch whole wheat tortilla; ½ cup pineapple juice; 2 cups water; coffee/tea

LUNCH
EAT OUT! Thai restaurant: Order chicken lettuce wraps; Fresh fruit cup; 2 cups water; tea/other non-caloric beverage

DINNER
Italian-Style Tilapia (p. 262); Small salad: 1 cup mixed greens + sliced radishes + 1 tbsp chopped parsley + 1 small tomato, sliced + Simple Dressing*; 2 cups water; tea/other non-caloric beverage

DAY 9

BREAKFAST
Omelette: In a nonstick pan, cook 1 egg + 1 tbsp chopped green pepper + 1 tbsp chopped cilantro + 2 tbsp salsa; 1 slice whole grain toast; ½ cup orange juice; 2 cups water; coffee/tea

LUNCH
Large tuna salad: 2 oz fresh grilled or canned tuna + 2 cups mixed greens + ½ cup steamed green string beans + 3 red onion slices + 3 cherry tomatoes + Simple Dressing*; 4–6 (½ oz) low-fat whole wheat crackers or crispbreads; 1 cup mixed berries; 2 cups water; tea/other non-caloric beverage

DINNER
Chicken veggie stir-fry (see tip): Sauté 3 oz chicken + 3 cups of mixed vegetables, sliced + 2 tsp peanut oil + 2 tsp minced garlic + ½ tsp sesame seeds + 1 tbsp low-sodium soy sauce + ½ tsp sesame oil (add at end of cooking); ⅓ cup brown rice; 2 cups water; tea/ other non-caloric beverage

DAY 10

BREAKFAST
½ cup cottage cheese mixed with 2 tbsp shredded carrot + 2 tbsp chopped cucumber + 2 tbsp shredded broccoli stalk or celery + 1 tbsp chopped parsley, salt and pepper to taste; 1 slice whole-grain toast; ½ cup pineapple juice; 2 cups water; coffee/tea

LUNCH
EAT OUT! Vietnamese restaurant: Order sweet and sour fish stew + 2 fresh vegetable salad rolls; Fresh fruit cup; 2 cups water; tea/other non-caloric beverage

DINNER
Lamb chops and greens: 3 oz grilled lamb chops + 1 cup roasted Brussels sprouts (tossed in ½ tsp EVOO); 1 cup winter squash or ½ cup yam; Large salad: 2 cups mixed greens + ½ cup sliced cucumber + ¼ cup sliced mushrooms + ¼ cup diced red pepper + 1 tbsp diced avocado + Simple Dressing*; 2 cups water; tea/other non-caloric beverage

DAY 11

BREAKFAST
Egg foo young omelette: In a nonstick pan cook 1 egg + 2 tbsp chopped scallions + ¼ cup mung bean sprouts + ¼ cup sliced mushrooms + ⅓ cup brown rice + ½ tsp low-sodium soy sauce; ½ cup orange juice; 2 cups water; coffee/tea

LUNCH
Tuna salad sandwich: 2 oz tuna + 1 dill pickle, finely chopped + ¼ tsp minced ginger + ¼ tsp curry powder + 1 tsp reduced-fat mayonnaise + lettuce leaves on 2 slices whole grain bread; sliced mixed vegetables on the side; 1 cup cubed melon; 2 cups water; tea/other non-caloric beverage

DINNER
Turkey with veggies: 3 oz roast turkey (light or dark meat) + 1 cup roasted Brussels sprouts (tossed in ½ tsp EVOO) + ½ cup roasted red pepper, sliced ; ½ cup baked yam or 1 cup winter squash; Large salad: 1 cup mixed greens + 1 cup raw spinach + ½ cup mung bean sprouts + 3 cherry tomatoes + 1 tbsp chopped Italian parsley + Simple Dressing*; 2 cups water; tea/other non-caloric beverage

DAY 12

BREAKFAST
Omelette: In a nonstick pan, cook 1 egg + 1 tbsp chopped green pepper and 1 tbsp chopped cilantro + 2 tbsp salsa; 1 slice whole-grain toast; ½ cup orange juice; 2 cups water; coffee/tea

LUNCH
EAT OUT! Subway: Order any 6-inch "Fresh Fit" sub on the menu (limit condiments to vinegar, salt and pepper) OR order any "Fresh Fit for Kids" sub + apple slices; 2 cups water; Tea/other non-caloric beverage OR **Chicken sandwich:** 2 oz sliced grilled chicken breast or deli chicken + lettuce leaves and tomato slices + 3 avocado slices + mustard on 2 slices of whole-grain bread; mixed greens salad + Simple Dressing; apple; 2 cups water; tea/other non-caloric beverage

DINNER
Spicy Orange Beef & Broccoli (p. 261); Large salad: 2 cups mixed greens + 6 sliced radishes + 1 tbsp fresh chopped parsley + 1 tbsp chopped red pepper + Simple Dressing*; 2 cups water; tea/other non-caloric beverage

DAY 13

BREAKFAST
1 egg prepared any way; 1 slice whole-grain toast topped with 1–2 tbsp plain yogurt, sliced tomato and cucumber; ½ fresh grapefruit; 2 cups water; coffee/tea

LUNCH
Chicken sandwich: 2 oz grilled, sliced chicken breast or deli chicken + lettuce leaves and tomato slices + 3 avocado slices + mustard on 2 slices of whole-grain bread; Mixed greens salad + Simple Dressing*; 1 apple; 2 cups water; tea/other non-caloric beverage

DINNER
EAT OUT! Japanese restaurant: Order 6 pieces of sushi (with rice) + seaweed salad + cucumber sunomono (a small vinegar-based salad) + miso soup; 2 cups water; tea/other non-caloric beverage

DAY 14

BREAKFAST
½ cup cooked oatmeal + ½ cup plain nonfat Greek yogurt + 2 tbsp dried fruit; 2 cups water; coffee/tea

LUNCH
Turkey salad: 2 oz sliced turkey breast + 2 cups mixed greens + 1 stalk chopped celery + ½ cup broccoli florets + 1 tbsp toasted sunflower seeds + Simple Dressing*; 4–6 (½ oz) low-fat whole wheat crackers or crispbreads; 1 orange; 2 cups water; tea/other non-caloric beverage

DINNER
Roasted chicken with Kale Chips: 3 oz roasted chicken + 2 cups Kale Chips (p. 222); ½ cup steamed parsnips or baked potato; Large salad: 2 cups mixed greens + ½ cup steamed green string beans + 3 red onion rings + 3 cherry tomatoes + Simple Dressing*; 2 cups water; tea/other non-caloric beverage

Workouts

As briefly mentioned earlier, you will have five or six training sessions each week. At least three of these sessions should be cardio, and two or three should be with weights (This chapter contains an At-Home Workout starting on p. 32). Here are a few different workout options for you to choose from.

5-Day Plans

MONDAY: 60 minutes cardio
TUESDAY: 45 minutes weights
WEDNESDAY: 60 minutes cardio
THURSDAY: 45 minutes weights
FRIDAY: 60 minutes cardio

MONDAY: 30–45 minutes weights, 30 minutes cardio
TUESDAY: 60 minutes cardio
WEDNESDAY: 30–45 minutes weights, 30 minutes cardio
THURSDAY: 60 minutes cardio
FRIDAY: 30–45 minutes weights, 30 minutes cardio

6-Day Plans

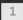

MONDAY: 60 minutes cardio
TUESDAY: 45 minutes weights
WEDNESDAY: 60 minutes cardio
THURSDAY: 45 minutes weights
FRIDAY: 60 minutes cardio
SATURDAY: 45 minutes weights

MONDAY: 30–45 minutes weights, 30 minutes cardio
TUESDAY: 60 minutes cardio
WEDNESDAY: 30–45 minutes weights, 30 minutes cardio
THURSDAY: 60 minutes cardio
FRIDAY: 30–45 minutes weights, 30 minutes cardio
SATURDAY: 60 minutes cardio

Don't feel limited to 60 minutes for cardio; if you want to do more then go ahead, but you don't have to. Make sure you are challenging yourself. Have goals you are working toward every workout and every week. For example, on Monday you managed five minutes jogging on the treadmill without having to walk. On Wednesday, see if you can manage six minutes, or even five minutes and 30 seconds. Last week you used eight-pound dumbbells for biceps curls. This week you can try for 10 pounds, even if it's only for part of your set.

These changes sound small, and perhaps they are, but they add up, and that is how we progress. Having these constant goals also makes working out more fun! For more about motivation and goal setting, see page 146.

All About Cardio

You may hear the term "cardio" and not know where it came from or what it really means. In a nutshell, cardio gets its name because it strengthens your cardiovascular system. Your cardiovascular system is made up of your heart, lungs, veins and arteries. Throughout your entire life, blood is continuously pumping through this system, providing nutrients (including oxygen) to every tiny cell in your body. The engine driving this whole system is your heart and you could say the energy provider for the engine is your lungs.

When you do cardio exercise, your lungs expand more and you breathe more heavily because your cells are screaming for more oxygen. Your heart then pumps faster in order to get that oxygen to those cells. The end result once cardio becomes a regular part of your life is that your heart and lungs get stronger and more efficient.

"Great," you say, "but what does this have to do with me losing weight?" Plenty! Cardiovascular exercise burns calories, and that helps a great deal with weight loss. Weight training builds muscle, which helps keep your metabolism in high gear, but cardio burns more calories while you do it. To reap all of the calorie-burning and metabolism-boosting rewards, your best bet is to follow a program that includes both cardio and weight training.

Turn the page for a list of some popular forms of cardiovascular exercise, and the approximate calories they burn per hour.

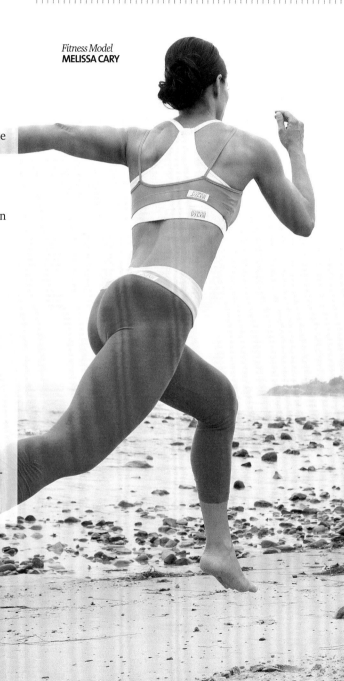

Fitness Model
MELISSA CARY

ACTIVITY, EXERCISE OR SPORT	CALORIES BURNED PER HOUR			
	130 LB	155 LB	180 LB	205 LB
Cycling, <10 mph, leisure bicycling	235	280	325	370
Cycling, 10–11.9 mph, light	355	420	490	560
Cycling, 12–13.9 mph, moderate	470	565	655	745
Cycling, 14–15.9 mph, vigorous	590	705	815	930
Cycling, 16–19 mph, very fast, racing	710	845	980	1115
Stationary cycling, very light	175	210	245	280
Stationary cycling, light	325	385	450	510
Stationary cycling, moderate	415	495	570	650
Stationary cycling, vigorous	620	740	860	975
Circuit training, minimal rest	470	565	655	745
Stair climber	530	635	735	840
Rowing machine, light	205	245	285	325
Rowing machine, moderate	415	495	570	650
Rowing machine, vigorous	500	600	695	790
Rowing machine, very vigorous	710	845	980	1115
Ski machine	415	495	570	650
Aerobics, low impact	295	350	410	465
Aerobics, high impact	415	495	570	650
Aerobics, step aerobics	500	600	695	790
Running, 5 mph (12 minute mile)	470	565	655	745
Running, 6 mph (10 minute mile)	590	705	815	930
Running, 7 mph (8.5 minute mile)	680	810	940	1070
Running, 8 mph (7.5 minute mile)	795	950	1105	1255
Running, 9 mph (6.5 minute mile)	885	1055	1225	1395
Running, 10 mph (6 minute mile)	945	1125	1310	1490
Running up stairs	885	1055	1225	1395
Jumping rope, fast	710	845	980	1115
Jumping rope, moderate	590	705	815	930
Jumping rope, slow	470	565	655	745
Roller skating	415	495	570	650
In-line skating	415	495	570	650

ACTIVITY, EXERCISE OR SPORT	CALORIES BURNED PER HOUR			
	130 LB	155 LB	180 LB	205 LB
Squash	710	845	980	1115
Tennis	415	495	570	650
Hiking, with backpack	415	495	570	650
Hiking, cross country	355	420	490	560
Race walking	385	455	530	605
Rock climbing, mountain climbing	470	565	655	745
Walking, < 2.0 mph, very slow	120	140	165	185
Walking 2.0 mph, slow	150	175	205	235
Walking 3.0 mph, moderate	195	230	270	305
Walking 3.5 mph, brisk pace	225	265	310	355
Walking 3.5 mph, uphill	355	420	490	560
Walking 4.0 mph, very brisk	295	350	410	465
Walking 5.0 mph	470	565	655	745
Kayaking	295	350	410	465
Swimming laps, freestyle, fast	590	705	815	930
Swimming laps, freestyle, slow	415	495	570	650
Water aerobics, water calisthenics	235	280	325	370
Water jogging	470	565	655	745
Ice skating, average speed	415	495	570	650
Ice skating, rapid	530	635	735	840
Cross country skiing, slow	415	495	570	650
Cross country skiing, moderate	470	565	655	745
Cross country skiing, vigorous	530	635	735	840
Cross country skiing, uphill	975	1160	1350	1535
Snow skiing, downhill skiing, light	295	350	410	465
Downhill snow skiing, moderate	355	420	490	560
Elliptical, moderate	560	675	800	885
Snowshoeing	470	565	655	745

Calculations are based on research data from Medicine & Science in Sports & Exercise, *and are rounded to the nearest five calories.*

Notice that the harder you work at a specific exercise the more energy you use to perform it and, ultimately, the more fat you burn. Most cardio machines have charts that show heart rate zones, suggesting where your heart rate should be for fat burning and cardio, but these charts are misleading. When you exercise at a lower intensity you burn a higher percentage of fat, but the energy (calories) you burn is higher the more intensely you exercise. The most effective heart rate for fat loss is the highest heart rate you can stay at for a minimum of 20 minutes, but it's even better if you can stay at it for 30 to 60 minutes.

The exception to this is interval training, which is a very effective way to burn fat and improve your cardiovascular fitness. The idea behind interval training is that you can increase your fitness level much more quickly if you work very hard – hard enough that you cannot continue for an extended period of time – and combine those intense periods with easy periods. During the easy periods your heart rate decreases and your breathing comes under control, allowing you to recover enough for another intense period.

Interval training increases your fitness level quickly and helps to burn extra fat, but you must use this form of training judiciously – it can lead you to an overtrained state, in which your body cannot recover enough before you stress it again. When you are overtrained, your nervous system becomes taxed and you do not make the physical gains you should. Do interval training no more than twice per week at an absolute maximum, and space those workouts as far apart as possible, to get the most gains with the least risk.

Keep in mind that the level you exercise at depends on your present fitness level. If you already exercise regularly and have good cardio fitness and strength, then you can work at a much more advanced level. If your biggest form of exercise in the past six months has been walking to your car, then you will want to start much more slowly and ease your way into it.

FIT TIP

"My treadmill is right next to my bed so when I wake up I have no excuses for not getting my cardio done first thing in the morning."

– *Felicia Romero, fitness model*

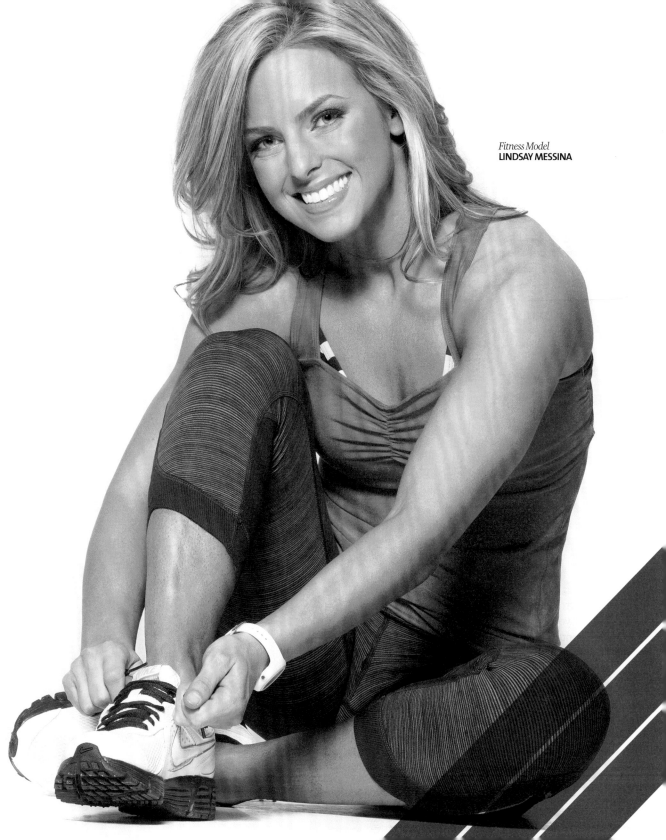

Fitness Model
LINDSAY MESSINA

Your At-Home Workout

No gym? No problem! For this routine, all you will need are a couple of dumbbells – inexpensive and easily available at your local sports store, Walmart or maybe even a thrift shop. After warming up, perform 2 sets of 15 reps for each of the following moves.

Warmup

Before hitting these resistance moves, you'll need to get your body warmed up with about five minutes of easy cardio. You have many options: You can use a treadmill, exercise bike or elliptical if you have one. Otherwise you can skip, do jumping jacks, dance or even go for a brisk walk outside for a few minutes. Once you're warmed up, you can start your resistance moves.

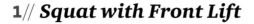

1// *Squat with Front Lift*

TONES THESE AREAS:
LEGS, GLUTES, SHOULDERS

SET UP/ Stand straight with your feet six to eight inches apart and hold a light dumbbell in each hand. Your palms should face the front of your thighs **[A]**.

ACTION/ Raise your arms to shoulder height. Lift weights up until your arms are parallel to the floor **[B]**. Lower your arms, then immediately bend your legs to squat toward the floor **[C]**. When your thighs are almost level with the floor, press through your heels to return to the start. Repeat, alternating lifts and squats.

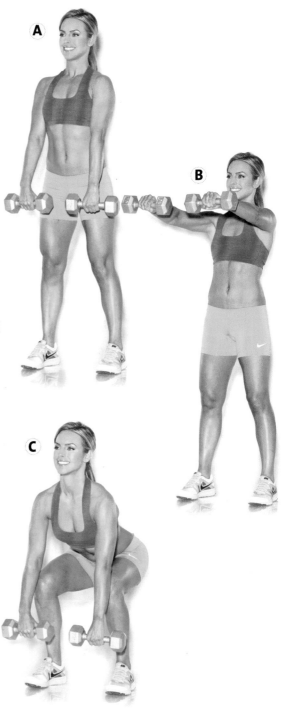

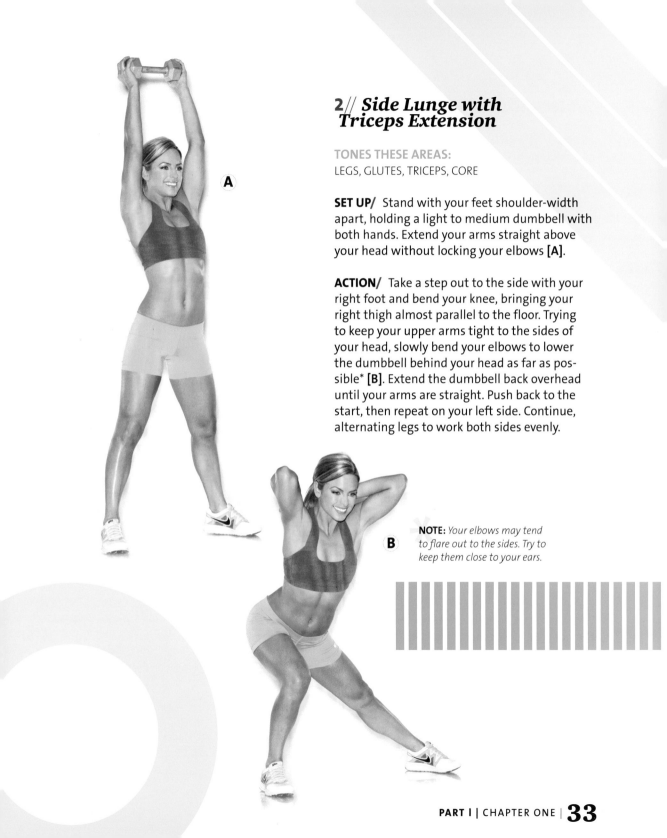

2// Side Lunge with Triceps Extension

TONES THESE AREAS:
LEGS, GLUTES, TRICEPS, CORE

SET UP/ Stand with your feet shoulder-width apart, holding a light to medium dumbbell with both hands. Extend your arms straight above your head without locking your elbows **[A]**.

ACTION/ Take a step out to the side with your right foot and bend your knee, bringing your right thigh almost parallel to the floor. Trying to keep your upper arms tight to the sides of your head, slowly bend your elbows to lower the dumbbell behind your head as far as possible* **[B]**. Extend the dumbbell back overhead until your arms are straight. Push back to the start, then repeat on your left side. Continue, alternating legs to work both sides evenly.

NOTE: *Your elbows may tend to flare out to the sides. Try to keep them close to your ears.*

3// *Deadlift with Row*

TONES THESE AREAS:
GLUTES, HAMSTRINGS, BACK, CORE

SET UP/ Stand with your feet spaced six to eight inches apart. Hold a medium dumbbell in each hand at your sides with your palms facing your thighs [A].

ACTION/ Bend forward at your waist until your torso is almost parallel to the floor, or slightly higher, letting your arms hang down past your knees [B]. Using your back, pull both weights up toward the sides of your rib cage [C], then slowly lower them back down. Return to the starting position, then repeat.

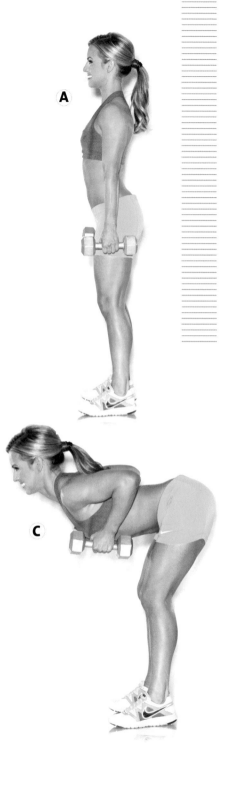

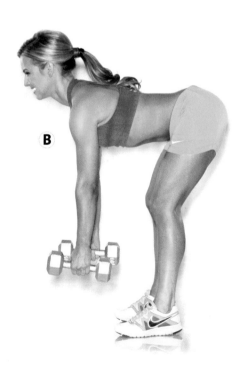

4// *Lunge*

TONES THESE AREAS:
LEGS, GLUTES

SET UP/ Stand with your feet spaced six to eight inches apart. Hold a dumbbell in each hand at your sides with your palms facing your thighs **[A]**.

ACTION/ Take a big step forward with your left foot, dropping your right knee almost to the floor, making sure to stand straight and tall while doing so **[B]**. Push off with your left foot, bringing it back to the starting position. Repeat with right leg.

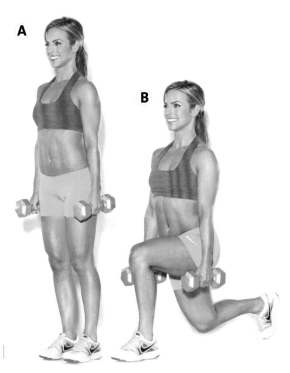

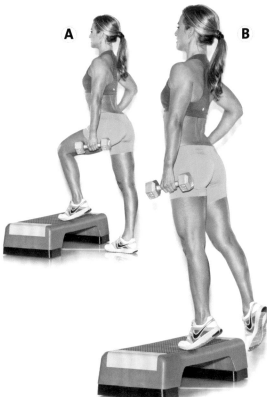

5// *Calf Raise on Step*

TONES THESE AREAS:
CALVES

SET UP/ Step onto a stair or other step, holding a weight in the hand of the same side as the foot you step up with **[A]**.

ACTION/ Lift up onto your toes. If you have a wall or banister close by you can touch it lightly for support **[B]**. Lower your heel way down to get a good stretch before lifting back up on your toes for the next rep. Switch the weight to the other hand and repeat on opposite side.

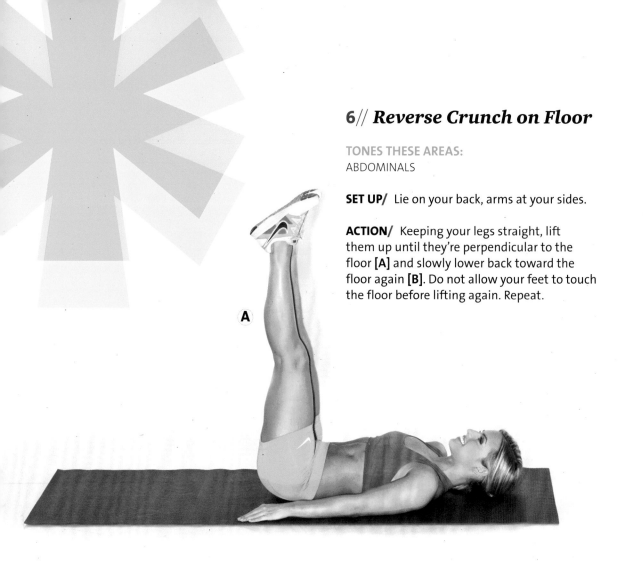

6// *Reverse Crunch on Floor*

TONES THESE AREAS:
ABDOMINALS

SET UP/ Lie on your back, arms at your sides.

ACTION/ Keeping your legs straight, lift them up until they're perpendicular to the floor **[A]** and slowly lower back toward the floor again **[B]**. Do not allow your feet to touch the floor before lifting again. Repeat.

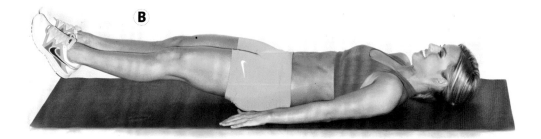

7 // *Plank*

TONES THESE AREAS:
ABDOMINALS AND LOWER BACK

SET UP/ Get in a full pushup position up on your toes, but keep your forearms on the floor **[A]**.

ACTION/ Hold this position, making sure your body is in a straight line from your feet to your shoulders. Don't allow your rear to sink down or stick up. Hold for as long as possible.

ADVANCED/ Do a side plank **[B]**. Make sure your feet are stacked and your body is in a straight line. This is great for your obliques and transverse abdominis.

ALTERNATIVE/ Try doing a plank on an exercise ball **[C]**.

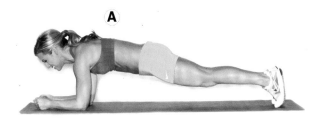

A

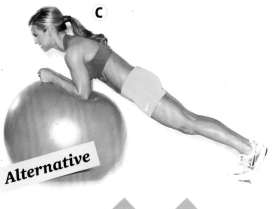

C

Alternative

Advanced

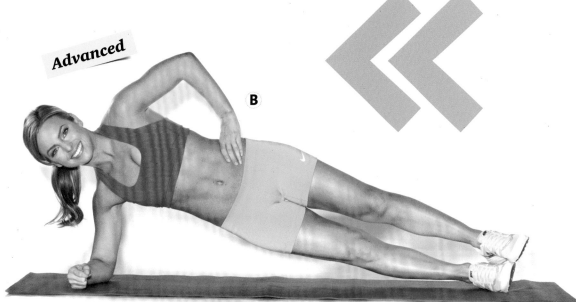

B

The oxygen Diet Solution Success *Story*

"I reached all my fitness goals!"

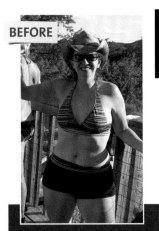

BEFORE

BEFORE: 220 lb

NOW: 112 lb

AGE: 34

HEIGHT: 5'2"

LOCATION: Austin, Texas

OCCUPATION: Mom of three boys

FAVORITE BODY PART: Legs

Kelly Smith has never loved bra shopping. Weighing in at 220 pounds at her heaviest, the last thing she wanted to do was stand half-naked in front of a mirror. But not anymore. Now more than 100 pounds lighter, she recalls a recent Victoria's Secret shopping spree, where the saleswoman complimented her on an "athletic" physique. "No one has ever called me that before!"

Fighting Cellulite

For Kelly, losing the weight wasn't the problem. She got down to 125 pounds by tightening up her diet. But what should have been a "woohoo!" moment was overshadowed by leftover cellulite. "Every time I left the house, I felt as if a giant spotlight was highlighting my legs!"

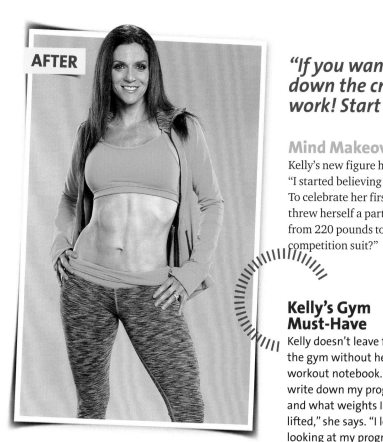

AFTER

"If you want a tight body, put down the creams — none of them work! Start building muscle!"

Mind Makeover

Kelly's new figure has brought her a new outlook: "I started believing in myself in my everyday life." To celebrate her first figure competition, Kelly threw herself a party. "How many moms can go from 220 pounds to standing on stage in a tiny competition suit?"

Kelly's Gym Must-Have

Kelly doesn't leave for the gym without her workout notebook. "I write down my program and what weights I lifted," she says. "I love looking at my progress!" To personalize her journal, she even draws little faces next to each workout, representing her mood.

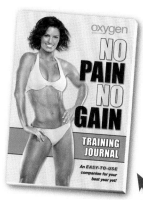

Order your *Oxygen No Pain No Gain Training Journal* today!
1-888-254-0767

Tightening Up

Kelly committed to a mix of cardio and strength sessions each week. No longer relying on a low calorie count to see results, she steered toward clean eating and learned an important lesson: "I was shocked to see that in order to maintain a lean body, I had to eat a lot of food – and not just carrots and celery," she says. Kelly also found the secret cellulite weapon: track workouts three times a week and weightlifting with none other than fitness model Monica Brant. "Monica coaching me keeps me running strong on the track," she says.

Party Ready

"I love the fact that my body is now party ready seven days a week. If someone calls and wants to go out that night, knowing I always have something to wear that fits well makes all the hard work worth it."

Daily Diet

Eating clean, fat-blasting foods was key to tightening up Kelly's body. Here's a sample of what's inside her fridge:

· Oatmeal

· Cottage cheese

· Asparagus

· Sweet potatoes

· Steak

· Brown rice

· Chicken breast

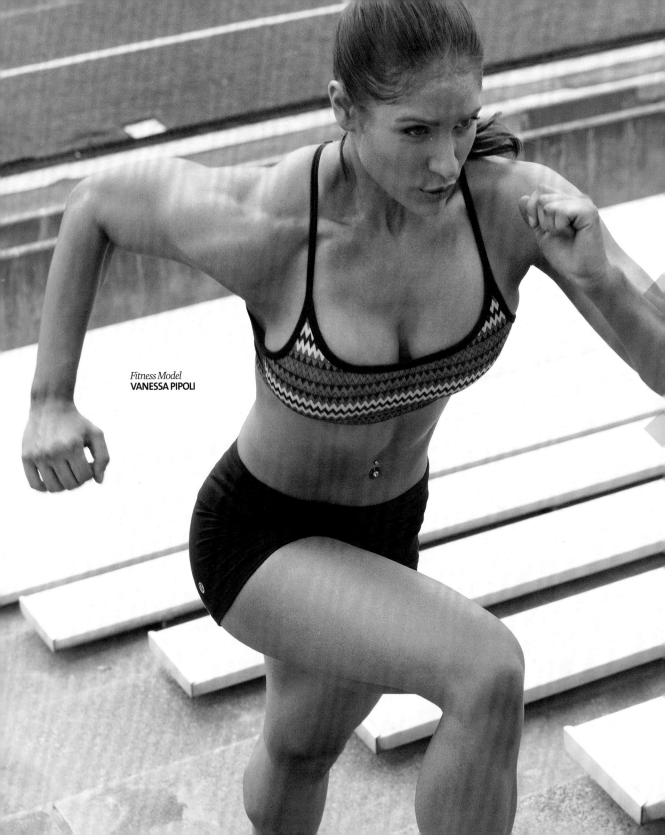

Fitness Model
VANESSA PIPOLI

Quick Fat-Loss Diet

Break through plateaus, get ready for an event or lose those last 10 pounds

We all know (or at least we all should know!) that it's best to lose weight slowly. Gradual weight loss is more likely to be permanent, less likely to lead to yo-yo dieting and is less likely to result in stretched skin. All this being said, however, we all have times when we want to lose a few pounds quickly for some event or another. Maybe you gained a few pounds over the holidays and are now panicking because you'll soon be going on a Caribbean cruise, or perhaps you've been invited to a pool party and want to look hot in your bikini. Whatever the reason, you want that weight gone – pronto!

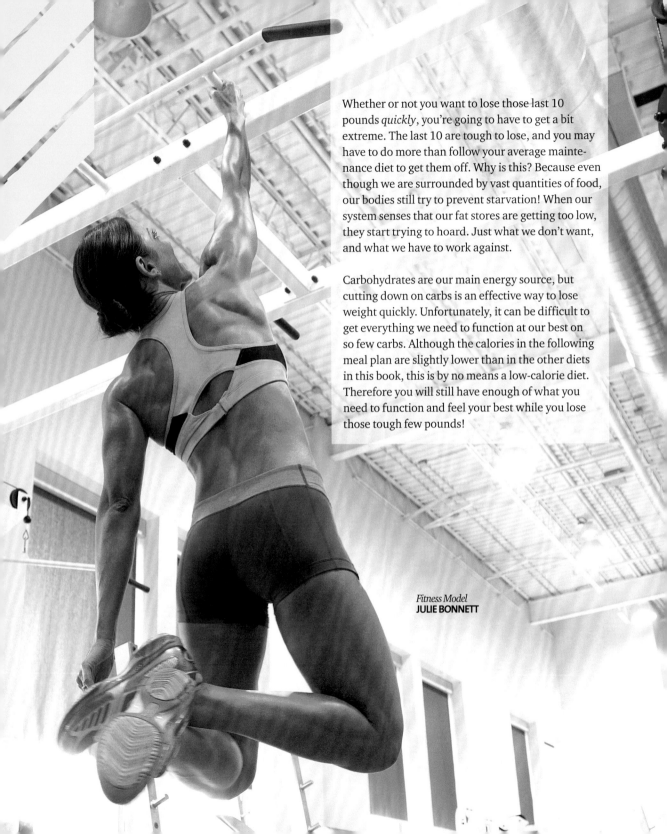

Whether or not you want to lose those last 10 pounds *quickly*, you're going to have to get a bit extreme. The last 10 are tough to lose, and you may have to do more than follow your average maintenance diet to get them off. Why is this? Because even though we are surrounded by vast quantities of food, our bodies still try to prevent starvation! When our system senses that our fat stores are getting too low, they start trying to hoard. Just what we don't want, and what we have to work against.

Carbohydrates are our main energy source, but cutting down on carbs is an effective way to lose weight quickly. Unfortunately, it can be difficult to get everything we need to function at our best on so few carbs. Although the calories in the following meal plan are slightly lower than in the other diets in this book, this is by no means a low-calorie diet. Therefore you will still have enough of what you need to function and feel your best while you lose those tough few pounds!

Fitness Model
JULIE BONNETT

Your Quick Fat-Loss Diet Meal Plan

While it's fine to follow this diet for 28 days, if you have more than 10 or 15 pounds to lose then it's in your best interest to follow The Basic *Oxygen* Diet instead (see p. 18).

If you hit a plateau while following one of the other diets in this book, you can hop on over here to the Quick Fat-Loss Diet for a couple of weeks to give your progress a bit of a jumpstart. Do keep in mind that if you stay on this diet for longer than 28 days, you could impact your weight loss in a negative way. This diet is 20 percent carbs, 40 percent protein and 40 percent fats.

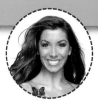
Snack Time!

In addition to the three meals per day listed in the Quick Fat-Loss Diet meal plan, you can have two daily snacks. These can be around exercise (one before and one after) or if you are not working out then one in the morning and one in the afternoon.

Optimally you will place the pre- and postworkout snacks exactly before and after you exercise, whenever that is during the day. However, if you exercise immediately after a meal or within 30 minutes of your next meal, move the pre- and/or postworkout snacks to another time during the day when a snack will break up a period of longer than three hours between meals.

SNACK 1:
- 1 cup plain low-fat Greek yogurt
- ½ cup fresh berries, halved
- ½ ounce (about 1 tbsp) slivered or sliced almonds

SNACK 2:
Smoothie – blend together:
- 1 cup nonfat milk
- ½ cup frozen berries
- 1 scoop (20 grams) whey protein isolate (look for one with no additives)

SWEET TREATS

Once per week, you can treat yourself with **one serving** of either one of these snacks (not both!). It should be consumed postworkout.

- Peppermint Protein Ice Cream (p. 273)
- Chocolate Power Pudding (p. 274)

For more tips on treats, see p. 183.

QUICK FAT-LOSS DIET MEAL PLAN

BEFORE YOU BEGIN:

Follow this meal plan twice for the 28-day plan.

If the variety of the plan has you feeling overwhelmed, you can choose a few of your favorites and then repeat them. You can swap one breakfast for another, or one lunch for another, or one dinner for another. But don't swap dinner for lunch, or breakfast for dinner and so on.

If absolutely necessary, you can also switch the order of meals within one day, but ideally you should not.

*

> *You will be having the Simple Dressing on an almost daily basis. For recipe, see p. 46.*
>
> ** *This fish dish can be substituted with the Grilled Raspberry Salmon on p. 266.*

DAY 1

BREAKFAST
Omelette: In a nonstick skillet, heat olive oil and cook 1 egg + 2 egg whites + 1 oz mozzarella cheese + 1 oz smoked salmon + 1 tbsp chopped chives or scallions + 2 tbsp diced tomato; 2 cups water; coffee/tea

LUNCH
Large salad: 2 cups mixed greens + ½ cup sliced cucumber + ¼ cup sliced mushrooms + ¼ cup diced red pepper + ¼ avocado, sliced + 5 green olives + 4 oz grilled chicken, sliced + 2 tbsp crumbled blue cheese (or 2 tbsp toasted pine nuts) + Simple Dressing*; 2 cups water; tea/other non-caloric beverage

DINNER
Ginger Salmon in Parchment Paper (p. 253); Large salad: 1 cup mixed greens + 1 cup raw spinach + ½ cup mung bean sprouts + 3 cherry tomatoes + 1 tbsp chopped Italian parsley + 1 tbsp toasted sliced almonds + Simple Dressing*; 2 cups water; tea/other non-caloric beverage

DAY 2

BREAKFAST
Frittata: Lightly sauté 1 tsp canola oil + 1 tbsp minced shallots + 2 tbsp shredded zucchini + 1 tbsp chopped red pepper + 1 egg + 2 egg whites, slightly beaten + 2 oz Canadian or turkey bacon; 2 cups water; coffee/tea

LUNCH
Chicken veggie stir-fry (see tip, p. 46): Sauté 4 oz chicken breast strips + 3 cups mixed vegetables, sliced + 1½ tbsp peanut oil + 2 tsp minced garlic + 1 tsp sesame seeds + 1 tbsp low-sodium soy sauce + ¼ tsp sesame oil (add at end of cooking); 2 cups water; tea/other non-caloric beverage

DINNER
Scallops or halibut cheeks with beets and greens: Lightly sauté 6 oz sea scallops or halibut cheeks + 1 tbsp olive oil + ½ tbsp minced garlic + couple of drops of truffle oil at end of cooking; steam 2 cups Swiss chard + 1 cup cubed golden or red beets + toss with 1 tsp olive oil and herbs; Large salad: 2 cups mixed greens + 6 radishes, sliced + 1 tbsp chopped parsley + 1 small tomato, sliced + Simple Dressing*; 2 cups water; tea/other non-caloric beverage

DAY 3

BREAKFAST
Egg foo young omelette: In a nonstick pan, heat 1 tsp canola oil and add 1 egg + 2 egg whites + 2 tbsp chopped scallions + ¼ cup mung bean sprouts + ¼ cup sliced mushrooms + ½ tsp low-sodium soy sauce; 2 cups water; coffee/tea

LUNCH
Large salad: 2 cups mixed greens + ½ cup steamed green string beans + 3 red onion slices + 3 cherry tomatoes + 5 green olives + 1 oz feta cheese, cubed + 4 oz fresh grilled or canned tuna + Simple Dressing*; 2 cups water; tea/other non-caloric beverage

DINNER
Halibut stir-fry: Sauté raw garlic + ½ cup mushrooms + 2 tbsp onions + 1 stalk chopped celery + 1 cup snow peas + 5 oz sliced halibut fillet seasoned with low-sodium soy sauce, ginger, and canola oil; Large salad: 1 cup shredded red and green cabbage + 1 cup shredded bok choy + ½ tsp toasted sesame seeds + Simple Dressing*; 2 cups water; tea/other non-caloric beverage

DAY 4

BREAKFAST
Egg and cottage cheese:
1 egg, prepared any way
+ ¾ cup cottage cheese
mixed with 2 tbsp
shredded carrot + 2 tbsp
chopped cucumber +
2 tbsp shredded broccoli
stalk or celery + 1 tbsp
chopped parsley; 2 cups
water; coffee/tea

LUNCH
EAT OUT! Vietnamese
restaurant: Order sweet
and sour fish stew +
sautéed vegetable dish;
2 cups water; tea/other
non-caloric beverage

DINNER
Lamb chops and greens:
6 oz grilled lamb chops
+ 1 cup roasted Brussels
sprouts tossed in EVOO
(extra-virgin olive oil);
Large salad: 2 cups mixed
greens + ½ cup sliced
cucumber + ¼ cup sliced
mushrooms + ¼ cup diced
red pepper + ¼ avocado,
sliced + 5 olives + Simple
Dressing*; 2 cups water;
tea/other non-caloric
beverage

DAY 5

BREAKFAST
Salmon and egg lettuce
rolls: 3 large iceberg
lettuce leaves + 2 oz
smoked salmon + 1 hard-
boiled egg + 2 egg whites
mixed with 1 tsp sugar-
free mayonnaise +
½ tsp yellow mustard; 2
cups water; coffee/tea

LUNCH
Chicken salad: 4 oz grilled
chicken breast, sliced +
2 cups mixed greens +
½ cup sliced cucumber +
¼ cup sliced mushrooms
+ ¼ cup diced red bell
peppers + ¼ avocado,
sliced + 5 green olives +
2 tbsp sunflower seeds +
Simple Dressing*; 2 cups
water; tea/other non-
caloric beverage

DINNER
Steak with olive tapenade
and cucumber:
5 oz grilled tenderloin +
½ cup sautéed mushrooms,
onions, 1½ cups chard +
EVOO and garlic; 2 tbsp
olive tapenade + ½ cup
sliced cucumber (spread
tapenade on cucumber
slices); **Large salad:**
1½ cups mixed greens +
6 radishes, sliced + 1 tbsp
fresh chopped parsley +
1 small tomato, sliced +
Simple Dressing*; 2 cups
water; tea/other non-
caloric beverage

DAY 6

BREAKFAST
Cucumber breakfast
canapés: 1 cucumber
sliced into ¼-inch-thick
disks, each disk topped
with ¼-inch-thick disks
sliced from 2 hard-boiled
eggs. Top disks with a
mixture of 2 oz ricotta
cheese whisked with salt
and pepper + ⅓ avocado,
mashed + 2 tsp lemon
juice + chopped cilantro;
2 cups water; coffee/tea

LUNCH
Tuna salad lettuce rolls:
4 oz tuna + ½–1 tbsp
sugar-free mayonnaise +
1 dill pickle, finely chopped
+ ¼ tsp minced ginger
+ ¼ tsp curry powder
combined and wrapped
in large iceberg lettuce
leaves; sliced mixed
vegetables on the side;
2 cups water; tea/other
non-caloric beverage

DINNER
Roasted chicken with Kale
Chips: 4 oz roasted chicken
+ 2 cups Kale Chips
(p. 222); **Large salad:**
2 cups of mixed greens +
½ cup steamed green
string beans + 3 red onion
rings + 3 cherry tomatoes +
5 green olives +
2 oz cheese, cubed +
Simple Dressing*;
2 cups water; tea/other
non-caloric beverage

DAY 7

BREAKFAST
Sausage with egg:
1 3-oz chicken sausage
(try Isernio's or any other
brand with 0 carbs) +
1 egg, prepared any way
you like + ⅓ avocado,
sliced and sprinkled with
lemon juice and salt;
2 cups water; coffee/tea

LUNCH
Easy & Elegant Tuna Bites
(p. 226); 2 cups water; tea/
other non-caloric beverage

DINNER
Sirloin burger with caprese
salad: 5 oz broiled sirloin
burger + 12 asparagus
spears tossed with minced
garlic and grilled; layer
together 1 medium
tomato, sliced + 2 oz fresh
mozzarella cheese, sliced
+ fresh basil leaves +
drizzle with EVOO + 1 tsp
balsamic vinegar; **Large
salad:** 2 cups greens +
½ cup cauliflower florets
+ 5 green olives + 1 tbsp
fresh chopped parsley +
Simple Dressing*; 2 cups
water; tea/other non-
caloric beverage

QUICK FAT-LOSS DIET MEAL PLAN

SIMPLE DRESSING

You will be eating a large salad almost every day topped with this fat-blasting vinaigrette mix.

1 tbsp extra virgin olive oil

2 tsp red wine vinegar

Sea salt and pepper, to taste

Mix all ingredients in a small bowl or mason jar. Pour over salad. Makes 1 serving. You can make a larger batch and measure out one 1½-tbsp serving per salad.

Nutrients per serving:
Calories: 126, Total Fat: 14 g,
Saturated fat: 2 g, Trans Fat: 0 g,
Cholesterol: 0 mg, Sodium: 8.5 mg,
Total Carbohydrates: 0 g,
Dietary Fiber: 0 g, Sugars: 0 g,
Protein: 0 g, Iron: 0 mg

STIR-FRY TIP

When a stir-fry recipe calls for mixed vegetables, feel free to use any combination of the following abs-firming picks: broccoli, onions, carrots, zucchini, red pepper, red cabbage, mushrooms, snow peas, water chestnuts and bean sprouts.

DAY 8

BREAKFAST
Blueberry Protein Crepes (p. 217); 2 oz Canadian or turkey bacon on the side; 2 cups water; coffee/tea

LUNCH
EAT OUT! Thai Restaurant: Order chicken lettuce wraps; 2 cups water; tea/other non-caloric beverage

DINNER
Chicken veggie stir-fry (see tip at left): Sauté 6 oz chicken + 3 cups sliced mixed vegetables + 1½ tbsp peanut oil + 2 tsp minced garlic + 1 tsp sesame seeds + 1 tbsp low-sodium soy sauce + ¼ tsp sesame oil; add at end of cooking; 2 cups water; tea/other non-caloric beverage

DAY 9

BREAKFAST
Omelette: 2 eggs + 2 egg whites + 1 oz shredded cheddar cheese + ¼ avocado, sliced + 1 tbsp no-added-sugar salsa; 2 cups water; coffee/tea

LUNCH
Large tuna salad: 4 oz fresh grilled or canned tuna + 2 cups mixed greens + ½ cup steamed green string beans + 3 red onion slices + 3 cherry tomatoes + 5 green olives + 1 oz feta cheese, cubed + EVOO; 2 cups water; tea/other non-caloric beverage

DINNER
"Spaghetti" with meatballs: Sauté 2 cups spaghetti squash, shredded + 5 oz meatballs + ¼ cup mushrooms + ½ cup zucchini + garlic + olive oil + ½ cup organic, canned, chopped tomatoes in liquid or sauce + grated Parmesan cheese (optional); **Large salad:** 2 cups mixed greens + 6 sliced radishes + 1 tbsp fresh chopped parsley + 1 small tomato, sliced + Simple Dressing*; 2 cups water; tea/other non-caloric beverage

DAY 10

BREAKFAST
Egg and cottage cheese: 1 egg, prepared as you like + ¾ cup cottage cheese with 2 tbsp shredded carrot + 2 tbsp chopped cucumber + 2 tbsp shredded broccoli stalk or celery + 1 tbsp chopped parsley; 2 cups water; coffee/tea

LUNCH
EAT OUT! Vietnamese restaurant: Order sweet and sour fish stew + Sautéed vegetable dish; 2 cups water; tea/other non-caloric beverage

DINNER
Lamb chops with greens: 5 oz grilled lamb chops + 1 cup roasted Brussels sprouts, tossed in EVOO; **Large salad:** 2 cups mixed greens + ½ cup sliced cucumber + ¼ cup sliced mushrooms + ¼ cup diced red pepper + ¼ avocado, sliced + 5 olives + Simple Dressing*; 2 cups water; tea/other non-caloric beverage

DAY 11

BREAKFAST
Egg foo young omelette: 1 tsp canola oil + 1 egg + 2 egg whites + 2 tbsp chopped scallions + ¼ cup mung bean sprouts + ¼ cup sliced mushrooms + ½ tsp low sodium soy sauce; 2 cups water; coffee/tea

LUNCH
Tuna Salad: 4 oz fresh grilled or canned tuna + 2 cups leafy greens + ½ cup steamed green string beans + 3 red onion slices + 3 cherry tomatoes + 5 green olives + 1 oz feta cheese, cubed + EVOO; 2 cups water; tea/other non-caloric beverage

DINNER
Turkey or Pork with veggies: 5 oz roast turkey (light or dark meat) or pork chops + 1 cup roasted Brussels sprouts, tossed in EVOO + ½ cup roasted red pepper, sliced; Large salad: 1 cup mixed greens + 1 cup raw spinach + ½ cup mung bean sprouts + 3 cherry tomatoes + 1 tbsp chopped Italian parsley + 1 tbsp toasted sliced almonds + Simple Dressing*; 2 cups water; tea/other non-caloric beverage

DAY 12

BREAKFAST
Omelette: 2 eggs + 2 egg whites + 1 oz shredded cheddar cheese + ¼ avocado, sliced + 1 tbsp no-added-sugar salsa; 2 cups water; coffee/tea

LUNCH
EAT OUT! Subway: Order any of the protein-containing salads and request "double the protein."; 2 cups water; tea/other non-caloric beverage OR Turkey Salad: 4 oz sliced turkey breast + 2 cups greens + 1 stalk chopped celery + ½ cup broccoli florets + 2 cherry tomatoes + 1 tbsp toasted sunflower seeds + Simple Dressing*; 2 cups water; tea/other non-caloric beverage

DINNER
Speedy Scallops and Brussels Sprouts (p. 241); Large salad: 2 cups mixed greens + 6 sliced radishes + 1 tbsp chopped parsley + 1 small tomato, sliced + Simple Dressing*; 2 cups water; tea/other non-caloric beverage

DAY 13

BREAKFAST
Sausage with egg: 1 3-oz chicken sausage + 1 egg, prepared any way you like + ⅓ avocado, sliced and sprinkled with lemon juice and salt; 2 cups water; coffee/tea

LUNCH
Chicken salad: 4 oz grilled chicken breast, sliced + 2 cups leafy greens + ½ cup sliced cucumber + ¼ cup sliced mushrooms + ¼ cup diced red pepper + ¼ avocado, sliced + 5 green olives + 2 tbsp sunflower seeds + Simple Dressing*; 2 cups water; tea/other non-caloric beverage

DINNER
EAT OUT! Japanese restaurant: Order 6 oz sashimi + seaweed salad + cucumber sunomono (a small vinegar-based salad); 2 cups water; tea/other non-caloric beverage

DAY 14

BREAKFAST
Protein scramble: 1 egg + 2 egg whites + mushrooms and onions in light olive oil + 1 oz lox or other fish + 1 oz turkey sausage link or patty; 2 cups water; coffee/tea

LUNCH
Turkey Salad: 4 oz sliced turkey breast + 2 cups greens + 1 stalk chopped celery + ½ cup broccoli florets + 2 cherry tomatoes + 1 tbsp toasted sunflower seeds + Simple Dressing*; 2 cups water; tea/other non-caloric beverage

DINNER
Seared Ahi Tuna with Cilantro-Mint Raita (p. 265); Layer together 1 medium tomato, + 2 oz fresh mozzarella cheese slices + basil leaves + drizzle with Simple Dressing*; Large salad: 2 cups mixed greens + 6 radishes sliced + ¼ cup diced bell peppers + 1 tbsp fresh chopped parsley + Simple Dressing*; 2 cups water; tea/other non-caloric beverage

Your Fat-Blasting Workout

Farmer's Walk Complex

Perplexed by the word "complex?" Simply put, it's a string of exercises completed back to back without rest, using the same piece of equipment. This workout alternates four strength moves with two farmer's walk variations – a hip walk, in which you carry two dumbbells by your sides, and a shoulder walk, wherein you lift and hold the weights above your shoulders. These complexes are perfect for fostering fat loss while maintaining muscle as they elevate your heart rate, kick up your intensity and hit all your major muscle groups from head to toe.

But what exactly makes this workout so effective? "Farmer's walk complexes are high intensity, they involve the entire body and they demand extended repetitive effort," says Nick Tumminello, CPT, owner of Performance University in Baltimore, Maryland. "In short, the combination of these three factors will burn a ton of calories both during and postworkout, something that morning stroll on the treadmill simply can't match."

Proceed with Care

Even though this is a speedy routine and the moves may appear basic, these are challenging combinations that could potentially lead to injury if you are not careful. Keep in mind that this workout is suitable for intermediate to advanced fitness enthusiasts. Don't try this program until you have a few solid months of strength-training experience behind you. Start with the cardio/weight-training routine and schedule in The Basic *Oxygen* Diet chapter (p. 26). Also, it's a good idea to get familiar with the moves by first trying each exercise on its own to make sure you've got your form down pat.

Next, you need to gear up. To reduce your risk of injury while still pushing your body to its limits, grab a set of dumbbells that is the heaviest weight you can tolerate for your weakest exercise. Clear a straightaway that is 20 to 25 yards long – about a quarter of a football field or 20 to 25 big steps – and mark each end of the distance or find visual cues in the area that you can use; this will be your point A and point B. Make sure the terrain is flat and clear of debris.

As you do your complexes, make sure that you don't drop the weights without looking in order to save time – after all, slamming a dumbbell directly on your toes can sideline you from all activity for quite some time. If you have a stopwatch handy, great – it can help you keep time, as your rounds should be no more than three minutes in length.

Get to Work

Make sure your body is prepped and fully warmed up before beginning; try walking on a small incline for five to 10 minutes before starting this routine. To start, perform all reps of the first exercise at point A. Then carry the dumbbells as listed in the subsequent farmer's walk to point B and back to point A. Follow with the next exercise at point A and continue in the same manner until all exercises are completed before setting the dumbbells down to rest.

Follow the guidelines laid out in "Set Up Your Perfect Complex," on the facing page, to determine how many complexes to complete and how much rest you should aim for. Remember, this workout should be speedy but controlled: Time yourself each round to see if you need to kick it up a notch.

Set Up Your Perfect Complex

If you are new to the farmer's walk complex:

- Complete one full round of the sequence below
- Rest for up to three minutes
- Repeat a second time

After a few weeks, try increasing your intensity by:

- Adding another circuit, working up to four rounds in total
- Reducing your rest periods between rounds
- Increasing the repetitions for each exercise
- Increasing the weight used

FIT TIP

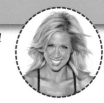

"I always brew a cup of flavored tea right before I sit down and eat. That way when my sweet tooth kicks in after the meal, I have something ready to help me avoid a temptation disaster!"

– Rita Catolino, fitness model and trainer to Tosca Reno

YOUR FARM-FRESH FAT ZAPPER

EXERCISE	REPS/DISTANCE
Squat and Press	12 reps
Farmer's Walk (hip carry)	40–50 yards total (20–25 yards up and back)
Plank Row (alternating arms)	10–16 reps total (5–8 reps per side)
Farmer's Walk (shoulder carry)	40–50 yards total (20–25 yards up and back)
Biceps Curl	8–12 reps per side
Repeat Farmer's Walk (hip carry)	40–50 yards total (20–25 yards up and back)

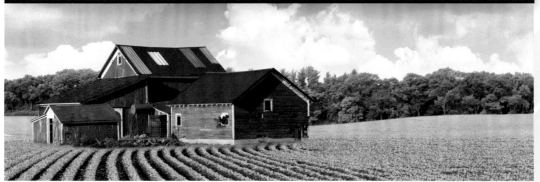

1// *Squat and Press*

TARGET MUSCLES:
QUADRICEPS, GLUTES, ANTERIOR DELTOIDS

SET UP/ Stand with your feet shoulder-width apart, toes pointing forward. Hold a dumbbell in each hand and raise your arms to bring the dumbbells directly above your wrists, upper arms slightly higher than shoulder height **[A]**.

ACTION/ Bend your knees to lower into a squat **[B]**. When your thighs are parallel to the ground, press through your heels to return to standing. At the same time, extend your arms above your head until they are straight but un-locked **[C]**. Slowly lower your arms back to the starting position and repeat.

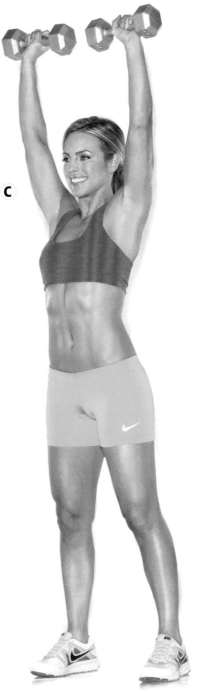

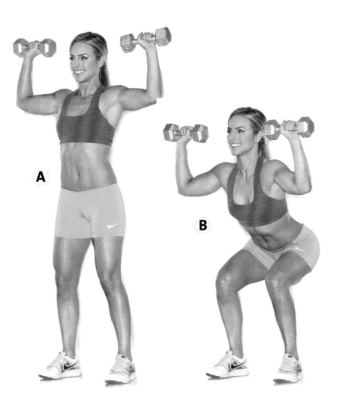

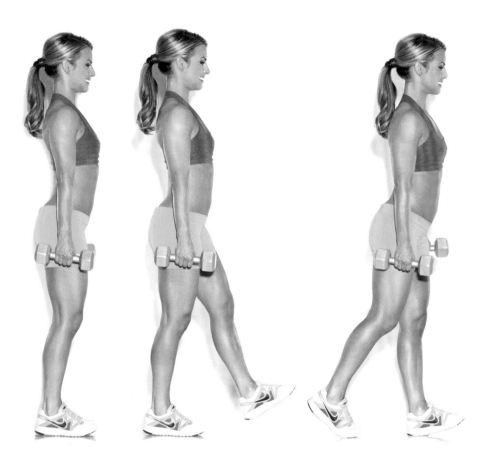

2// *Farmer's Walk (Hip Carry)*

TARGET MUSCLES:
QUADRICEPS, GASTROCNEMIUS, GRIP MUSCLES

SET UP/ Stand at your predetermined point A with your feet hip-width apart, holding a dumbbell in each hand with your arms extended by your sides.

ACTION/ Keeping your shoulder blades retracted and your eyes focused forward, take quick steps to bring yourself to point B. Without stopping, turn and make your way back to point A. Immediately move on to the next exercise in your complex.

FIT TIP

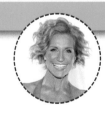

"You have to find the driving passion that will make you get your butt up off your chair and into motion."

– *Tosca Reno, author, motivational speaker and fitness model*

3// *Plank Row*

TARGET MUSCLES:
TRANSVERSE ABDOMINIS, LATISSIMUS DORSI, ANTERIOR DELTOIDS (SHOULDERS)

SET UP/ Get into a push-up position on the ground, gripping a dumbbell in each hand directly under your shoulders **[A]**. Space your legs shoulder-width apart or wider if you need additional support.

ACTION/ Using a smooth, controlled motion, pull one dumbbell up until it reaches the outside of your rib cage **[B]**. While your torso will naturally twist as you row, try to keep your shoulders as level as possible. Return the dumbbell to the ground, then repeat with your opposite arm, ensuring that you perform the same amount of reps on each side during your set.

ALTERNATIVE/ Make it even better! Do a push-up before each rep!

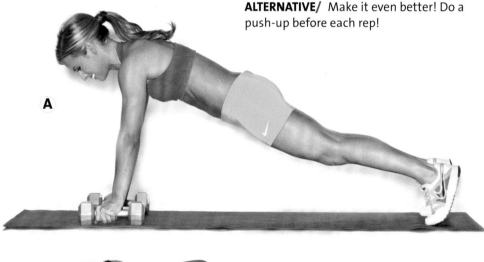

A

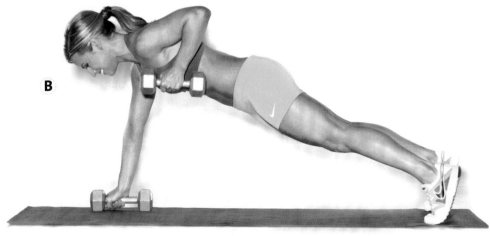

B

4// *Farmer's Walk (Shoulder Carry)*

TARGET MUSCLES:
QUADRICEPS, GASTROCNEMIUS, ANTERIOR DELTOIDS (SHOULDERS)

SET UP/ Hold a dumbbell in each hand at shoulder height with your arms bent, elbows pointing forward with palms facing in **[A]**. Make sure there is enough space between your arms so that you can see your path in front of you.

ACTION/ Walk toward point B using a swift gait **[B]**. Immediately turn and return to point A maintaining the same speed, then move on to your next exercise.

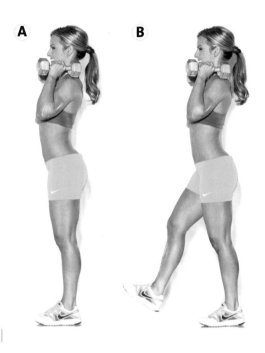

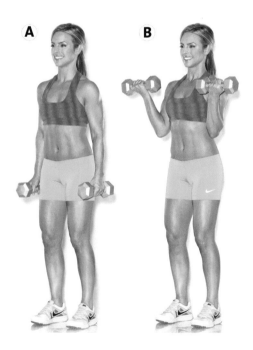

5// *Biceps Curl*

TARGET MUSCLES:
BICEPS

SET UP/ Stand with your feet hip-width apart, grasping a dumbbell in each hand **[A]**.

ACTION/ Bending your arms, bring the dumbbells to your shoulders **[B]**. Keep your upper arms close to your sides. Maintain a higher speed than you would when completing curls during your regular routine. You can also alternate your arms, but be careful not to use body momentum to get the dumbbells up.

The oxygen Diet Solution Success Story

WITH AN ARSENAL OF BEAT BOXING AND SILLY HUMOR, ABBY HUOT TOOK ON THE FITNESS STAGE AND CONQUERED HER FEAR OF FAILURE.

"I was the ultimate underdog!"

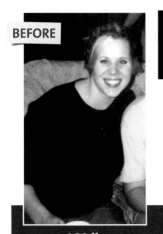

BEFORE

BEFORE: 190 lb
NOW: 138 lb
AGE: 30
HEIGHT: 5'6"
LOCATION: Lake Elmo, MN
OCCUPATION: Document control clerk
FAVORITE EXERCISE: Deadlifts

Surrounded by "serious" competitors backstage during fitness shows, Abby Huot likes to break the ice with a little humor. "What's wrong with doing the chicken dance to shake off some nerves?" says the 30-year-old, who's also been known to attempt beat boxing behind the curtain. "When I loosen up and get silly, it makes things way more fun."

Fish out of water

When it comes to pushing past the uncomfortable, Abby's a pro. A swimmer for over a decade, she felt intimidated the first day she tip-toed into the weight room at her gym. Everything was new and scary. "I was the ultimate underdog," she says. "I stuck out like a sore thumb." To overcome her crippling fear of failure, Abby decided she would have to fake it to make it.

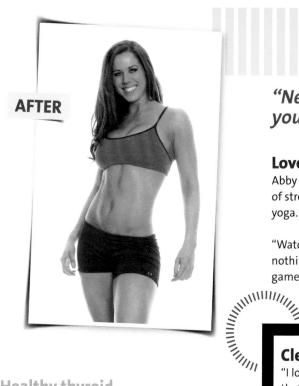

AFTER

"Never let someone else define your success or failure for you."

Love For The Game

Abby trains six days a week with a combination of strength training, cardio (including sprints) and yoga. But her secret athletic passion?

"Watching baseball and softball!" she says. "There's nothing better in the summer than an evening ball game in Minnesota!"

Healthy thyroid

Last year, Abby was diagnosed with a thyroid disorder (hypothyroidism), which had led to symptoms of fatigue and weight gain. Between medication from her doctor, proper sleep and her new fitness regimen, however, Abby now feels better and more energetic than ever.

Confidence counts

Sizing herself up against other women in the gym was Abby's biggest mental obstacle. "It's like they took all the girls in sports bras and tiny shorts and put them in there!" she says. As she got into the groove of her workouts and put on lean muscle, Abby slowly built up her confidence.

Pushing past limits

With over 10 competitions under her belt now, Abby still confronts her fears with a mix of audacity and laughter. "It doesn't matter how much tanner or sparkle you put on me before a show," she says, "I will always be the sarcastic dork in a suit. Life is so much more fun when you don't take it so seriously all the time."

Cleaning Up Her Act

"I look back and facepalm myself for thinking that chicken alfredo was healthy because it had chicken!" she says. Now, Abby sticks with a clean diet for success. Some of her favorite combinations:

BREAKFAST: Omelette made with goat cheese, spinach and diced red pepper

LUNCH: Stir-fry made with chicken and veggies

DINNER: Ahi tuna steak with sweet potatoes and asparagus

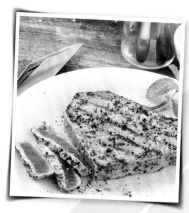

SNACKS BETWEEN MEALS: Dates, almonds, shakes

CHECK OUT p. 257 and p. 265 for two *Oxygen*-approved ahi tuna recipes!

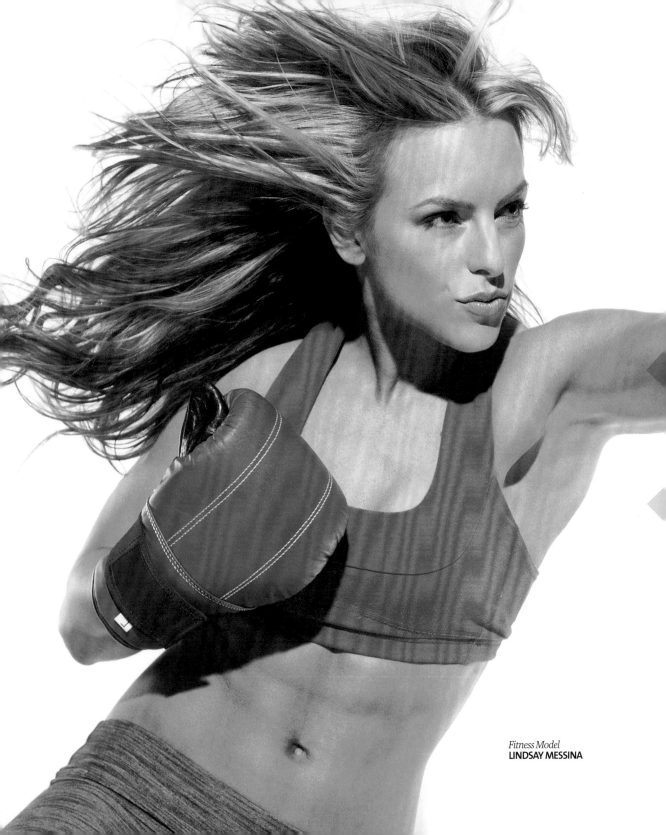

Fitness Model
LINDSAY MESSINA

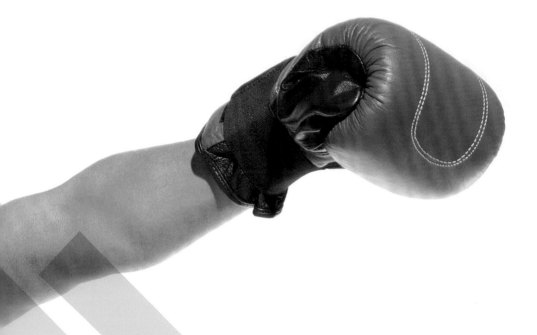

Super-Energy Diet

Power to get you through even the longest days

You bounce out of bed before your alarm clock goes off, dance around the kitchen while making breakfast for the family and whistle your way to work, where you breeze through the day, taking your lunch hour to go for a run or a spin class and then sail through afternoon meetings. After your nutritious homemade dinner, you drop the kids off at their respective sports practices and go for a samba lesson with your husband.

Does the previous paragraph sound like your day? No? Maybe you're more like the typical American who pushes snooze a few times before groggily stumbling around, pouring some cereal for the kids and yawning your way through your daily activities, buoyed by coffee and maybe a sugary snack or two.

What if you could find all the energy you needed to do everything you want each day? There's no end to what you could accomplish! Well, you can find that energy by following the diet and exercise plan in this chapter, along with the following tips.

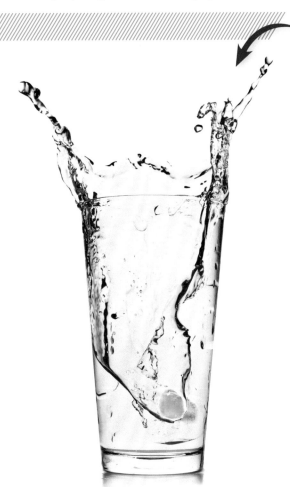

POWER UP!
10 Ways to Supercharge Your Energy

1 / Get enough sleep!
At *Oxygen* we often hear from women looking for some magic way to have more energy and when we ask them how much they sleep they seem surprised that it might matter. It *does* matter! The Mayo Clinic recommends seven to nine hours per night for the average adult.

2 / Drink water.
Every reaction that happens inside your body requires water, and if there isn't enough water, then everything from cell replication to digestion will require more effort.

3 / Get regular exercise.
It's a downward spiral – when you have no energy you don't want to exercise, but exercise actually revitalizes you. Make yourself do it and you'll have lots more energy afterward.

4 / Walk around.
Sitting for long periods of time zaps you. If you have to sit for your job, make sure to get up regularly and take a walk or stretch. If possible, it's great to break up your day of sitting with a lunchtime workout.

5 / Stick to a schedule.

Go to sleep at the same time and wake up at the same time each day, even on weekends. That way your internal clock will know exactly when it should be active and when to wind down.

6 / Avoid sugar, limit caffeine.

These are artificial forms of energy that lift you up and then make you crash and reach for more.

7 / Lose that extra weight.

It takes a lot of energy to lug those extra pounds around each day! Even an extra five or 10 pounds can make the simple act of going up a flight of stairs feel like a chore.

8 / Have more sex.

It makes you feel good and it's fun! There's a reason the man in that Viagra ad is happily skipping down the street in the morning.

9 / Have fun!

Don't take life too seriously – it will only weigh you down. Make an effort to look on the bright side of things. Dance around. Laugh. Play more.

10 / Limit alcohol use.

Save your drinking for the weekend, don't have more than two drinks at a time and never during the day. Alcohol is a depressant, and leaves you with little energy.

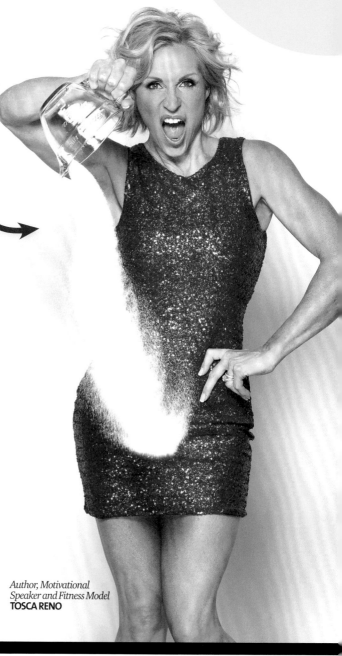

Author, Motivational Speaker and Fitness Model
TOSCA RENO

Your Super-Energy Diet Meal Plan

Another key way to gain energy is to eat regularly throughout each day. Start with a good breakfast and continue with nutritious meals and snacks all day long. Lucky for you, the following Super-Energy Diet will help you do just that. It offers 50 percent carbohydrates, since carbs are your main daily energy source, along with 25 percent protein and 25 percent fat. These regular meals will keep your energy level high throughout the day.

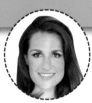
Snack Time!

In addition to the three meals per day listed in the Super-Energy Diet meal plan, you can have two daily snacks. These can be around exercise (one before and one after) or if you are not working out, then one in the morning and one in the afternoon.

Optimally you will place the pre- and postworkout snacks exactly before and after you exercise, whenever that is during the day. However, if you exercise immediately after a meal or within 30 minutes of your next meal, move the pre- and/or postworkout snacks to another time during the day when a snack will break up a period of longer than three hours between meals.

SNACK 1
- 1 cup plain low-fat yogurt (not Greek)
- ½ cup fresh berries, halved
- ½ ounce (about 1 tbsp) slivered or sliced almonds

SNACK 2
Smoothie – blend together:
- 1 cup nonfat milk
- ½ fresh banana (frozen is best)
- ½ cup frozen berries
- ½ scoop (10 grams) whey protein isolate (look for one with no additives)

SNACK 3
- One serving of Almond Butter Whey Cookies (p. 270)

SWEET TREATS

Once per week, you can treat yourself with **one serving** of only one of these snacks:

Preworkout
- Mini Chocolate Soufflés (p. 269)

Postworkout
- Peppermint Protein Ice Cream (p. 273)
- Chocolate Power Pudding (p. 274)

For more tips on treats, see p. 183.

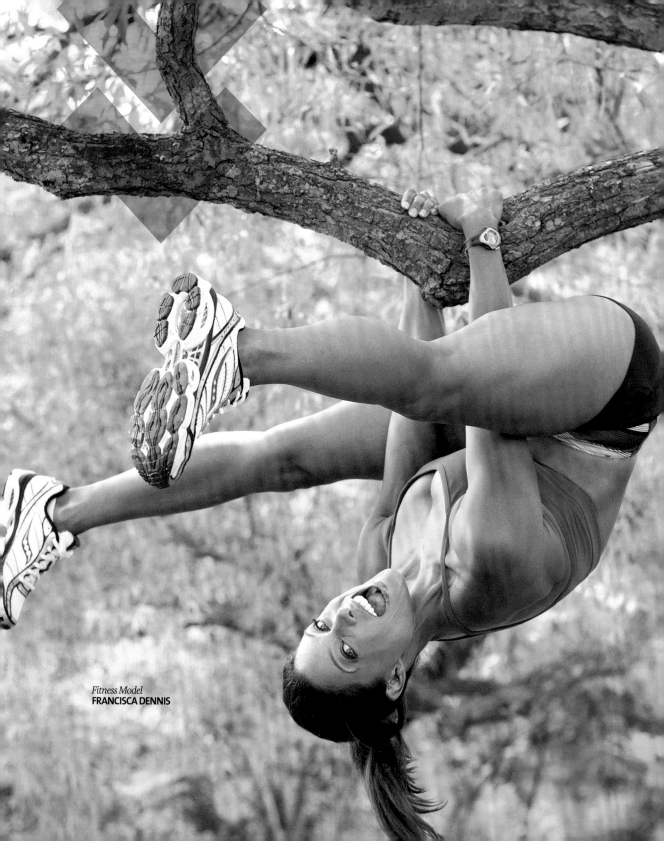

Fitness Model
FRANCISCA DENNIS

BEFORE YOU BEGIN:

Follow this meal plan twice for the 28-day plan.

If the variety of the plan has you feeling overwhelmed, you can choose a few of your favorites and then repeat them. You can swap one breakfast for another, or one lunch for another, or one dinner for another. But don't swap dinner for lunch, or breakfast for dinner and so on.

If absolutely necessary, you can also switch the order of meals within one day, but ideally you should not.

* *You will be having the Simple Dressing on an almost daily basis. For recipe, see p. 64.*

** This fish dish can be substituted with the Grilled Raspberry Salmon on p. 266.

DAY 1

BREAKFAST
Omelette: In a nonstick pan, cook 1 egg + 1 tbsp chopped onions or scallions + 2 tbsp diced tomato; ⅔ cup cooked steel-cut oats; 2 tbsp yogurt, any type; 2 tbsp dried fruit; ½ cup orange juice; 2 cups water; coffee/tea

LUNCH
Chicken Mango Salad Sandwich (p. 237); mixed greens salad + Simple Dressing*; 2 cups water; tea/other non-caloric beverage

DINNER
Grilled fish: 3 oz grilled fish of your choice, seasoned with 1 tsp EVOO (extra-virgin olive oil) + ½ tbsp lemon juice, sea salt, pepper; 12 asparagus spears grilled with crushed garlic; **Large salad:** 1 cup mixed greens + 1 cup raw spinach + ½ cup mung bean sprouts + 3 cherry tomatoes + 1 tbsp chopped Italian parsley + Simple Dressing*; ½ cup cooked quinoa; 2 cups water; tea/other non-caloric beverage

DAY 2

BREAKFAST
Egg tortilla: In nonstick pan, lightly sauté 1 tbsp minced shallots + 2 tbsp shredded zucchini + 1 tbsp chopped red pepper + 1 egg, slightly beaten. Divide egg mixture and 2 tbsp salsa between 2 6-inch whole wheat tortillas; 1 cup pineapple juice; 2 cups water; coffee/ tea

LUNCH
Chicken veggie stir-fry (see tip, p. 64): Sauté 2 oz chicken breast strips + 3 cups sliced mixed vegetables + 1½ tsp peanut oil + 2 tsp minced garlic + ½ tsp sesame seeds + 1 tbsp low-sodium soy sauce (add at end of cooking); ⅔ cup brown rice (**Leftover Tip:** Save ⅓ cup rice for tomorrow's breakfast); 1 orange; 2 cups water; tea/other non-caloric beverage

DINNER
Scallops (or other seafood) with beets and greens: Lightly sauté 1 tsp olive oil + ½ tbsp minced garlic + 3 oz sea scallops; steam 2 cups Swiss chard + 1 cup cubed golden or red beets + toss with herbs; ⅔ cup polenta; **Small salad:** 1 cup mixed greens + sliced radishes + 1 tbsp chopped parsley + 1 small tomato, sliced + Simple Dressing*; 2 cups water; tea/other non-caloric beverage

DAY 3

BREAKFAST
Egg foo young omelette: In a nonstick pan, cook 1 egg + 2 tbsp chopped scallions + ¼ cup mung bean sprouts + ¼ cup sliced mushrooms + ⅓ cup brown rice + ½ tsp low sodium soy sauce; 2 brown rice cakes with 1½ tbsp all-fruit spread; ½ cup orange juice; 2 cups water; coffee/tea

LUNCH
EAT OUT! Thai restaurant: Order chicken lettuce wrap; fresh fruit cup; 2 cups water; tea/other non-caloric beverage

DINNER
Ground Turkey & Pasta Primavera (p. 250); Large salad: 2 cups mixed greens + 6 sliced radishes + 1 tbsp fresh chopped parsley + 1 tbsp chopped red pepper + Simple Dressing*; 2 cups water; tea/other non-caloric beverage

DAY 4

BREAKFAST
½ cup cottage cheese mixed with 2 tbsp shredded carrot + 2 tbsp chopped cucumber + 2 tbsp shredded broccoli stalk or celery + 1 tbsp chopped parsley, salt and pepper to taste; 2 slices whole-grain toast with 1½ tbsp all-fruit spread; ½ cup pineapple juice; 2 cups water; coffee/tea

LUNCH
Anti-Stress Shrimp Salad (p. 229); Fresh fruit cup; 2 cups water; tea/other non-caloric beverage

DINNER
Lamb chops and greens: 3 oz grilled lamb chops + 1 cup roasted Brussels sprouts (tossed in ½ tsp EVOO and fresh lemon juice); 1 cup winter squash or ½ cup yam; **Large salad:** 2 cups mixed greens + ½ cup sliced cucumber + ¼ cup sliced mushrooms + ¼ cup diced red pepper + 1 tbsp diced avocado + Simple Dressing*; 2 cups water; Tea/other non-caloric beverage

DAY 5

BREAKFAST
Egg lettuce rolls: 2 large iceberg lettuce leaves + 1 hard-boiled egg, diced + 1 tbsp shredded carrot + 1 tbsp diced celery mixed with 1 tsp low-fat mayonnaise + ½ tsp mustard. Place ½ egg mixture onto each lettuce leaf and roll up; 1 cup cooked bulgur or ½ cup muesli with 1 cup fresh berries; ½ fresh grapefruit; 2 cups water; coffee/tea

LUNCH
Large salad: 2 cups mixed greens + ½ cup sliced cucumber + ¼ cup sliced mushrooms + ¼ cup diced red pepper + ⅓ cup diced avocado + 2 oz grilled chicken, sliced + Simple Dressing*; 4–6 (½ oz) low-fat whole wheat crackers or crispbreads; 1 apple; 2 cups water; tea/other non-caloric beverage

DINNER
Steak with olive tapenade and cucumber: 3 oz grilled tenderloin + ½ cup sautéed mushrooms, onions, 1½ cups chard + 1 tsp EVOO and garlic; 1 tbsp olive tapenade + ½ cup sliced cucumber (spread tapenade on cucumber slices); 2 cups winter squash or 1 cup yam; **Large salad:** 1½ cups mixed greens + sliced mixed veggies + fresh lemon juice, 1 tbsp Parmesan cheese + salt and pepper for dressing; 2 cups water; tea/other non-caloric beverage

DAY 6

BREAKFAST
1 egg prepared any way; 2 4-inch buckwheat pancakes with 1 cup fresh berries; ½ fresh grapefruit; 2 cups water; coffee/tea

LUNCH
Tuna salad sandwich: 2 oz tuna + 1 dill pickle, finely chopped + ¼ tsp minced ginger + ¼ tsp curry powder + 1 tsp low-fat mayonnaise + lettuce leaves on 2 slices of whole-grain bread; sliced mixed vegetables on the side; 1 cup cubed melon; 2 cups water; tea/other non-caloric beverage

DINNER
Roasted chicken with Kale Chips: 3 oz roasted chicken + 2 cups Kale Chips (p. 222); 1 cup steamed parsnips or baked potato; **Large salad:** 2 cups mixed greens + ½ cup steamed green string beans + 3 red onion rings + 3 cherry tomatoes + Simple Dressing*; 2 cups water; tea/other non-caloric beverage

DAY 7

BREAKFAST
Energizing Breakfast Wrap (p. 218); 2 cups water; coffee/tea

LUNCH
Veggie bean salad: 1 cup cooked beans (black, garbanzo, kidney, navy, pinto, white) + 2 cups leafy greens + 1 stalk chopped celery + ½ cup broccoli florets + 1 tbsp toasted sunflower seeds + Simple Dressing*; orange; 2 cups water; tea/other non-caloric beverage

DINNER
Sirloin burger (or meatless burger topped with soy cheese): 3 oz broiled sirloin or meatless burger with 1 oz soy cheese + lettuce, tomato, onion, mustard and 2 tsp ketchup on 1 whole-grain slider bun; 12 asparagus spears tossed with garlic and grilled; layer together 1 medium tomato, sliced + fresh basil leaves + drizzle with 1 tsp EVOO + 1 tsp balsamic vinegar; 1 cup "fries" from baking potato scrubbed, sliced into wedges, tossed with 1 tsp canola oil and baked; 2 cups water; tea/other non-caloric beverage

SIMPLE DRESSING

You will be eating a large salad almost every day topped with this fat-blasting vinaigrette mix.

1 tbsp extra virgin olive oil

2 tsp red wine vinegar

Sea salt and pepper, to taste

Mix all ingredients in a small bowl or mason jar. Pour over salad. Makes 1 serving. You can make a larger batch and measure out one 1½ Tbsp serving per salad.

Nutrients per serving:
Calories: 126, Total Fat: 14 g,
Saturated fat: 2 g, Trans Fat: 0 g,
Cholesterol: 0 mg, Sodium: 8.5 mg,
Total Carbohydrates: 0 g,
Dietary Fiber: 0 g, Sugars: 0 g,
Protein: 0 g, Iron: 0 mg

STIR-FRY TIP

When a stir-fry recipe calls for mixed vegetables, feel free to use any combination of the following abs-firming picks: broccoli, onions, carrots, zucchini, red pepper, red cabbage, mushrooms, snow peas, water chestnuts and bean sprouts.

DAY 8

BREAKFAST
Egg tortilla: In a nonstick pan, lightly sauté: 1 tbsp minced shallots + 2 tbsp shredded zucchini + 1 tbsp chopped red pepper + 1 egg, slightly beaten. Divide egg mixture and 2 tbsp salsa between 2 6-inch whole wheat tortillas; 1 cup pineapple juice; 2 cups water; coffee/tea

LUNCH
Shrimp & Corn Avocado Salad (p. 238); 1 cup mixed berries; 2 cups water; tea/other non-caloric beverage

DINNER
Scallops (or other seafood) with beets and greens: Lightly sauté 3 oz sea scallops + 1 tsp olive oil + ½ tbsp minced garlic; steam 2 cups Swiss chard + 1 cup cubed golden or red beets + toss with herbs; ⅔ cup polenta; **Small salad:** 1 cup mixed greens + sliced radishes + 1 tbsp chopped parsley + 1 small tomato, sliced + Simple Dressing*; 2 cups water; tea/other non-caloric beverage

DAY 9

BREAKFAST
Omelette: In a nonstick pan, cook 1 egg + 1 tbsp chopped onions or scallions + 2 tbsp diced tomato; ⅔ cup cooked steel-cut oats; 2 tbsp yogurt, any type; 2 tbsp dried fruit; ½ cup orange juice; 2 cups water; coffee/tea

LUNCH
Large tuna salad: 2 oz fresh grilled or canned tuna + 2 cups mixed greens + ½ cup steamed green string beans + 3 red onion slices + 3 cherry tomatoes + Simple Dressing*; 4–6 (½ oz) low-fat whole wheat crackers or crispbreads; 1 cup mixed berries; 2 cups water; tea/other non-caloric beverage

DINNER
Halibut stir-fry: Sauté raw garlic + ½ cup mushrooms + 2 tbsp onions + 1 stalk chopped celery + 1 cup snow peas + 3 oz sliced halibut filet seasoned with low-sodium soy sauce, ginger and 1 tsp canola oil in nonstick wok or pan; ⅔ cup cooked quinoa; **Large salad:** 1 cup shredded red and green cabbage + 1 cup shredded bok choy + Simple Dressing*; 2 cups water; tea/other non-caloric beverage

DAY 10

BREAKFAST
½ cup cottage cheese mixed with 2 tbsp shredded carrot + 2 tbsp chopped cucumber + 2 tbsp shredded broccoli stalk or celery + 1 tbsp chopped parsley, salt and pepper to taste; 1 slice whole-grain toast; ½ cup pineapple juice; 2 cups water; coffee/tea

LUNCH
Arugula Berry Salad with Steamed White Fish (p. 233); 2 cups water; tea/other non-caloric beverage

DINNER
Lamb chops and greens: 3 oz grilled lamb chops + 1 cup roasted Brussels sprouts (tossed in ½ tsp EVOO and fresh lemon juice); 1 cup winter squash or ½ cup yam; **Large salad:** 2 cups mixed greens + ½ cup sliced cucumber + ¼ cup sliced mushrooms + ¼ cup diced red pepper + 1 tbsp diced avocado + Simple Dressing*; 2 cups water; tea/other non-caloric beverage

DAY 11

BREAKFAST
Non-Fried Vegetable Quinoa (p. 234); 2 cups water; coffee/tea

LUNCH
Tuna salad sandwich: 2 oz tuna + 1 dill pickle, finely chopped + ¼ tsp minced ginger + ¼ tsp curry powder + 1 tsp low-fat mayonnaise + lettuce leaves on 2 slices whole-grain bread; sliced mixed vegetables on the side; 1 cup cubed melon; 2 cups water; tea/other non-caloric beverage

DINNER
EAT OUT! Japanese restaurant: Order chirashi sushi with rice + seaweed salad + cucumber sunomono (a small vinegar-based salad) + miso soup; 2 cups water; tea/other non-caloric beverage

DAY 12

BREAKFAST
Omelette: In a nonstick pan, cook 1 egg + 1 tbsp chopped onions or scallions + 2 tbsp diced tomato; ⅔ cup cooked steel-cut oats; 2 tbsp yogurt, any type; 2 tbsp dried fruit; ½ cup orange juice; 2 cups water; coffee/tea

LUNCH
Comforting Tuna Casserole (p. 258); 2 cups water; tea/other non-caloric beverage

DINNER
Chicken veggie stir-fry (see tip, p. 64): Sauté 3 oz chicken + 3 cups sliced mixed vegetables + 1 tsp peanut oil + 2 tsp minced garlic + 1 tbsp low-sodium soy sauce (add at end of cooking); ⅔ cup brown rice; 2 cups water; tea/other non-caloric beverage

DAY 13

BREAKFAST
1 egg prepared any way; 2 slices whole-grain toast topped with 2 tbsp yogurt and sliced tomato and cucumber; 1 cup fresh berries; ½ fresh grapefruit; 2 cups water; coffee/tea

LUNCH
Chicken sandwich: 2 oz grilled chicken breast, sliced or deli chicken + lettuce leaves and tomato slices + 3 avocado slices + mustard on 2 slices of whole-grain bread; **Small salad:** mixed greens + Simple Dressing*; apple; 2 cups water; tea/other non-caloric beverage

DINNER
Five-Spice Turkey (p. 249); **Large salad:** 1 cup mixed greens + 1 cup raw spinach + ½ cup mung bean sprouts + 3 cherry tomatoes + 1 tbsp chopped Italian parsley + Simple Dressing*; 2 cups water; tea/other non-caloric beverage

DAY 14

BREAKFAST
⅔ cup cooked steel-cut oats; ½ cup plain nonfat Greek yogurt; 2 tbsp dried fruit; ½ cup orange juice; 2 cups water; coffee/tea

LUNCH
EAT OUT! Subway: Order any 6-inch "Fresh Fit" sub on the menu (limit condiments to: vinegar, salt and pepper) OR order any "Fresh Fit for Kids" sub + apple slices; 2 cups water; tea/other non-caloric beverage OR Chicken sandwich: 2 oz grilled chicken breast, sliced or deli chicken + lettuce leaves and tomato slices + 3 avocado slices + mustard on 2 slices of whole-grain bread; **Small salad:** mixed greens + Simple Dressing*; apple; 2 cups water; tea/other non-caloric beverage

DINNER
Grilled Mussel Bruschetta (p. 225); **Roasted chicken with Kale Chips:** 3 oz roasted chicken + 2 cups Kale Chips (p. 222); 2 cups water; tea/other non-caloric beverage

Workouts

Our super energy workout is a plyometric workout. Plyometrics are very effective, very challenging, but also trying on the body. This workout should be performed twice per week. Then do regular cardio and weight training on the other days, to a maximum of six days per week. Here are some weekly options:

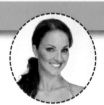
5-Day Plan

 1

MONDAY: Super-Energy Workout
TUESDAY: Weights
WEDNESDAY: Cardio
THURSDAY: Super-Energy Workout
FRIDAY: Weights

6-Day Plan

 1

MONDAY: Super-Energy Workout
TUESDAY: Cardio
WEDNESDAY: Weights
THURSDAY: Super-Energy Workout
FRIDAY: Cardio
SATURDAY: Weights

Your At-Home Workout

Warmup

Before beginning this program, warm up with some light cardio for five to 10 minutes. Move directly from one exercise to the next without resting. After completing the circuit once, rest for one to two minutes before beginning from the top. Repeat this circuit four or five times per workout.

NOTE: Do this plyo circuit in place of your regular cardio no more than twice per week, and always end with a thorough full-body cooldown and stretch session.

YOUR PLYO PLAN

PLYO MOVE	TIME
Jumping Lunge	30 seconds
180-Degree Squat	30 seconds
Lateral One-Legged Hop	1 minute
Bounding	1 minute

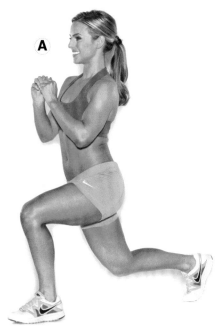

1// *Jumping Lunge*

Stand with your feet shoulder-width apart, hands on hips. Take a big step forward with one leg and bend both knees to lower your body toward the ground **[A]**.

When your forward leg forms a 90-degree angle, pause for one count before pushing off from the heel of your forward leg, propelling your body into the air **[B]**. When you're in mid-air, switch the positioning of your legs (front leg back, back leg forward), and land with soft knees, slowly lowering back toward the ground into a lunge **[C]**. Pause for one count before repeating.

Tip: Keep your front knee behind your toes.

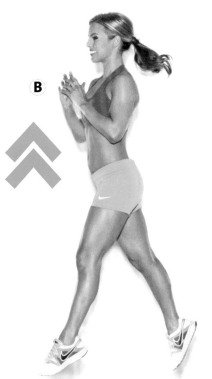

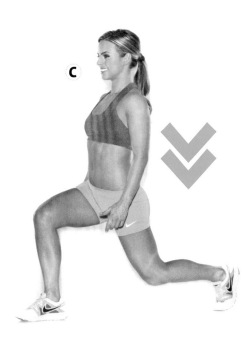

2// *180-Degree Squat*

Stand with your legs shoulder-width apart, arms extended naturally at your sides. Bend your knees to sink into a low squat, keeping your knees behind your toes at all times **[A]**.

Push through your heels to explode into the air, turning your body to face the opposite direction (180 degrees) **[B]** before landing with soft knees. Sink immediately into your squat position **[C]** and repeat.

Tip: Use your arms to help accelerate your speed and height when performing these squats.

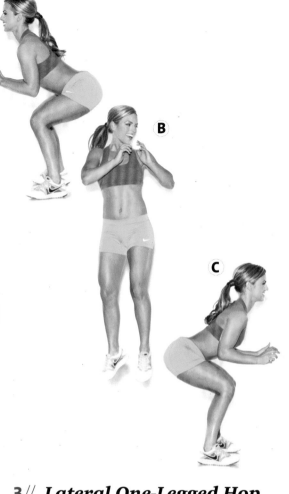

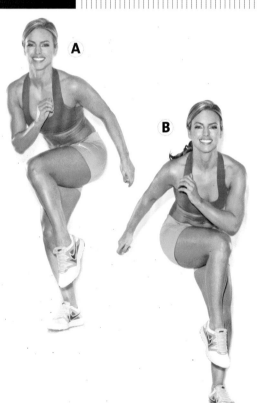

3// *Lateral One-Legged Hop*

Begin with feet shoulder-width apart, arms hanging naturally at your sides. Bend your left leg at the knee and raise it in front of your body until your thigh is parallel to the ground **[A]**. Pushing through your right heel, jump to the left, landing softly on your left foot as you bend your right knee, thigh parallel to the ground **[B]**. Repeat, moving back and forth from your right leg to your left leg.

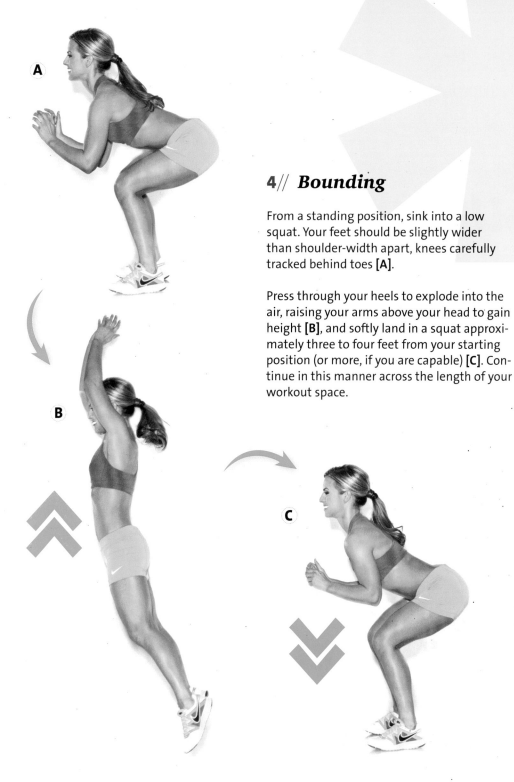

4// *Bounding*

From a standing position, sink into a low squat. Your feet should be slightly wider than shoulder-width apart, knees carefully tracked behind toes [A].

Press through your heels to explode into the air, raising your arms above your head to gain height [B], and softly land in a squat approximately three to four feet from your starting position (or more, if you are capable) [C]. Continue in this manner across the length of your workout space.

The oxygen Diet Solution
Success Story

DESPITE HER BUSY ON-THE-GO LIFESTYLE, ALISON HAGER LOST 92 POUNDS – AND KEPT THEM OFF!

"I gained a new respect for myself!"

BEFORE

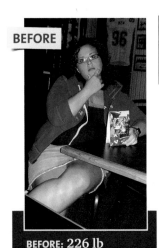

Before getting fit, Alison Hager had low self-esteem. In high school she weighed 226 pounds, and then repeatedly used yo-yo diets to drop and gain back the weight. But she didn't give up. In fact, she made it a point to do things the right way. "When I finally decided I was going to get healthy for good, I gained a new respect for myself," she says.

Race to health

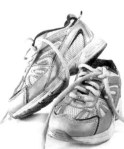

Recently, Alison completed a half-marathon – a far cry from her college days, when she needed four-hour afternoon naps just to have energy for homework. "Most of the time in college, I was dysfunctional. My mom said I was irritable and cranky." Then she was diagnosed with hypothyroidism in her senior year and began taking the appropriate medication. Now, Alison trains for her runs with interval cardio that includes sprints, jogs and walks, and she's seen her energy increase!

BEFORE: 226 lb
NOW: 134 lb
AGE: 23
HEIGHT: 5'5"
LOCATION: Beloit, KS
OCCUPATION: Teacher
FAVORITE EXERCISE: Walking lunges

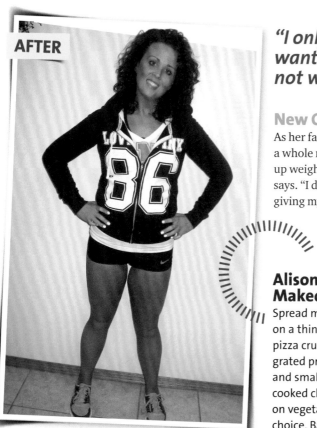

AFTER

"I only have one life to live. I want to live it to the fullest and not worry about my health."

New Outlook

As her fat-loss journey progressed, Alison developed a whole new outlook on health and fitness. "I gave up weighing and measuring myself for Lent," she says. "I decided to focus instead on eating clean and giving my all in each workout."

Alison's Pizza Makeover

Spread marinara sauce on a thin whole wheat pizza crust. Top with grated provolone cheese and small chunks of cooked chicken. Sprinkle on vegetables of your choice. Bake at 450°F for 12 minutes or until crust is crispy. Enjoy for lunch!

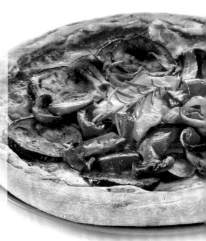

Core values

Diet was also important. "It was a huge transition going from comfort foods to healthier eating," she says, but planning her meals ahead of time helped. Now, Alison depends on foods that are easy to fix and transport (such as yogurt, fruit and whole wheat crackers). Lunchtime is also easy. "Brothy soups with vegetables keep me full longer."

Fit inspiration

When she first tried a plank, Alison lasted 15 seconds. Now, she nails a two-and-a-half-minute plank with ease. Down to 134 pounds, Alison has committed to an active way of life. "I know that it's a lifestyle change and that I'm not doing it for a number on the scale, but for my health."

Mixing It Up

To keep her body (and her mind) from getting bored, Alison mixes up her workouts with:

- Weight training
- Running
- Circuit training
- Plyometrics
- Zumba classes
- Suspension training

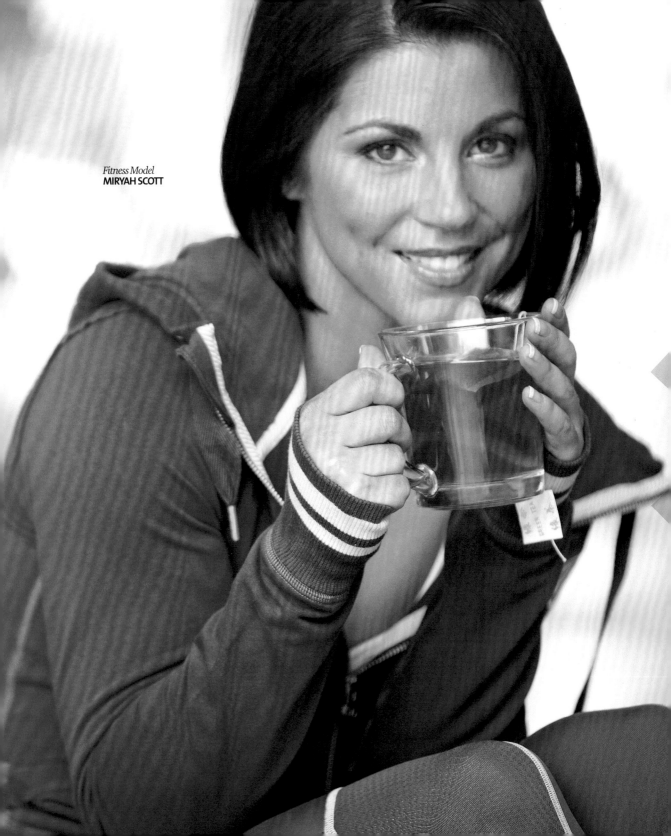

Fitness Model
MIRYAH SCOTT

Power-Immunity Diet

Build up your immune system

When you do your best to take good care of yourself, eat well and exercise regularly, getting sick can almost feel like an insult. Although no one can avoid getting sick indefinitely (even the most fervent users of hand sanitizers!), we all can certainly improve our body's ability to fight off illness – and that means everything from a mild flu or cold to a serious disease such as cancer. Your health is in your hands, and making small changes, such as the ones suggested in this chapter, can make a big difference.

We all have a working immune system – if we didn't we'd be forced to live like the famous "boy in the plastic bubble," cut off from the world and protected from all germs. But our immune systems function with varying degrees of ability. A person with AIDS, as an extreme example, might have a slightly depressed immune system or may have such a depressed immune system that he or she picks up any opportunistic disease encountered. A fairly healthy person will not see these extremes, but certainly some people seem to pick up every bug that crosses their path whereas others can take an extra vacation with all their unused sick days.

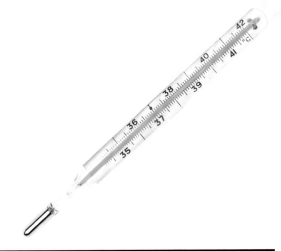

How can you fortify yourself against illness? According to Harvard Medical School, here are the most important ways to improve your immune system:

- Don't smoke.
- Eat a diet high in fruits, vegetables and whole grains, and low in saturated fat.
- Exercise regularly.
- Maintain a healthy weight.
- Control your blood pressure.
- If you drink alcohol, drink only in moderation.
- Get adequate sleep.
- Take steps to avoid infection, such as washing your hands frequently and cooking meats thoroughly.
- Get regular medical screening tests for people in your age group and risk category.

Having a consistently good diet and exercise plan is extremely beneficial, and the diet in this chapter in particular will help. At approximately 45 percent carbohydrates, 25 percent protein and 30 percent fat, this diet provides specific foods that encourage your immune system to work at its absolute peak. These foods provide a plethora of nutrients and anti-oxidants, and they are also anti-inflammatory.

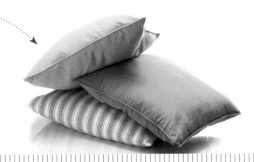

Why follow an anti-inflammatory diet?

Inflammation is an important part of our immune system response. When we have an injury or infection, the cells of that area release chemicals that begin the inflammatory response, which isolates the area and brings white blood cells to instigate the healing process. After the healing is complete, the inflammation ends. This is called acute inflammation. Chronic inflammation, however, is a dangerous condition whereby the chemicals that instigate inflammation are continuously released, keeping your body in a constant state of low-grade inflammation. We now know chronic inflammation is at least a factor in many (if not all) chronic diseases and conditions, from allergies to rheumatoid arthritis to heart disease and cancer.

Chronic inflammation may be caused by many factors in today's society, including pollution and household chemicals, but diet is also a major influence. If you eat lots of processed or refined foods along with red meat, you place yourself at huge risk of being in a state of chronic inflammation – and don't think this happens only as you age; even children can be in this state.

A diet rich in anti-inflammatory foods is extremely beneficial both for preventing chronic inflammation caused by diet and in helping to reduce the chances of chronic inflammation caused by external factors.

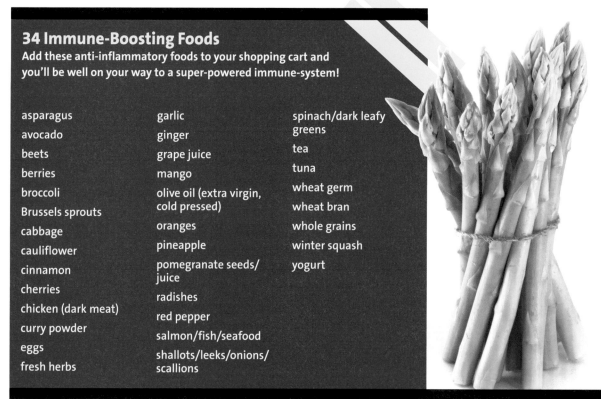

34 Immune-Boosting Foods

Add these anti-inflammatory foods to your shopping cart and you'll be well on your way to a super-powered immune-system!

asparagus
avocado
beets
berries
broccoli
Brussels sprouts
cabbage
cauliflower
cinnamon
cherries
chicken (dark meat)
curry powder
eggs
fresh herbs

garlic
ginger
grape juice
mango
olive oil (extra virgin, cold pressed)
oranges
pineapple
pomegranate seeds/juice
radishes
red pepper
salmon/fish/seafood
shallots/leeks/onions/scallions

spinach/dark leafy greens
tea
tuna
wheat germ
wheat bran
whole grains
winter squash
yogurt

Mighty Micronutrients

With the surplus of prepackaged foods and junk food, it's no surprise that the standard North American diet lacks the required amount of micronutrients. Fruits and vegetables have become runners-up to packaged and fast foods, which causes a deficiency in vitamins and minerals. Without these key micronutrients, our immune system weakens, our bodies become malnourished and we run into a whole mess of health problems. But this can easily be prevented! Here are some immune-boosting vitamins and minerals you should make sure to include in your diet.

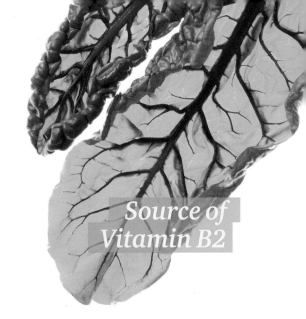

Source of Vitamin B2

Selenium

Selenium is a trace mineral that helps to build antioxidants in our bodies. A study from the University of Arizona Cancer Center suggests that people with low selenium levels are at greater risk of colon, lung and prostate cancers. Working alongside vitamin E, this mineral protects cell membranes from free-radical damage.

FIND IT IN: button mushrooms, cod, shrimp, tuna, halibut, salmon, mustard seeds, Brazil nuts

Vitamin A

Vitamin A plays a key role in the maintenance of good vision and skin. A deficiency in this vitamin can reduce the strength of your body's immunity and increase the risk of infectious disease. It can also cause night blindness and dry skin. A study from Kaiser Permanente Northern California concluded that vitamin A may reduce the risk of skin cancer.

FIND IT IN: carrots, squash, pumpkin and other yellow-orange fruits and vegetables, green leafy vegetables, liver and dairy products, cod and fish liver oils

Vitamin B2

Like vitamin A, vitamin B2 (aka riboflavin) helps maintain vision and skin health, and it plays an important role in the production of ATP, a molecule that transports energy in cells. A study conducted in Japan revealed that vitamin B2 enhances resistance to bacterial infections in mice, but it's unclear what that means for humans' immune response. However, studies indicate that riboflavin can reduce the instances of migraines, along with decreasing the risk of cataracts.

FIND IT IN: leafy greens, nuts, legumes, wheat germ, wild rice, mushrooms, organ meats (liver, kidney and heart)

Vitamin B6

Since vitamin B6 is important for the metabolism, immune and nervous system, as well as the creation of hormones and red blood cells, it's no wonder that a deficiency can weaken immune response. Some people choose to boost their B6 stores with supplements, but in most cases a healthy balanced diet will provide adequate amounts.

FIND IT IN: sunflower seeds, wheat germ, soybeans, walnuts, lentils, lima beans, buckwheat flour, bananas, avocados

Vitamin C

Since humans cannot manufacture vitamin C, it's essential we consume this vitamin to help boost immunity and antioxidants, and produce collagen to help us recover from wounds or surgery. This is why all our lives we've been told to take vitamin C to prevent colds. Vitamin C can also work with other micronutrients to provide benefits for the immune system.

FIND IT IN: bell peppers, papaya, kale, oranges, lemon juice, parsley, Brussels sprouts, strawberries

Vitamin D

The sunshine vitamin was rightly named, since our skin produces vitamin D when exposed to ultraviolet light from the sun. Vitamin D is needed to produce serotonin, the "feel-good" neurotransmitter in our brains, and it improves bone health. Researchers from the American Association for the Advancement of Science have found that vitamin D signals an anti-microbial response to the bacteria responsible for tuberculosis.

FIND IT IN: sunshine, orange juice, fortified dairy products, beef liver, eggs, fortified cereal, most fish and fish oil

Vitamin E

Vitamin E can be used to amp up the immune system. An important contributor to the production of B-cells, vitamin E helps to fight off unwanted bacteria. A significant deficiency of vitamin E can cause pain or numbness in the extremities, muscle weakness and impaired immune response. A study, from the USDA Human Nutrition Research Center on Aging at Tufts University, has shown that a higher intake of vitamin E can increase antibody responses to hepatitis B and tetanus after vaccination.

FIND IT IN: seeds, nuts, vegetable oils, grains, lentils

Zinc

This trace mineral is important for brain function, vision maintenance, sperm production and wound healing. Zinc is also essential for maintaining the immune system, where a deficiency can affect the ability of immune cells to function properly and increase the risk of infection. However, too much zinc can inhibit the function of the immune system altogether.

FIND IT IN: almonds, lima beans, chickpeas, yogurt, lentils, pumpkin and sesame seeds

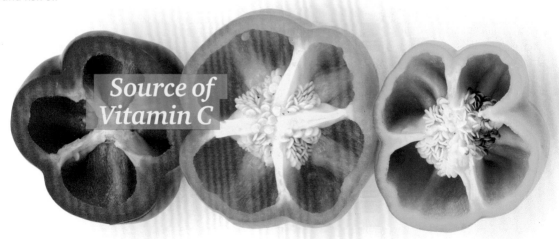

Source of Vitamin C

Your Power-Immunity Diet Meal Plan

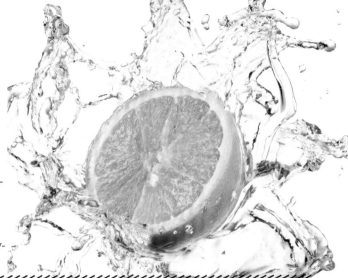

The key to all of the *Oxygen* diets, and this diet in particular, is the density of nutrients, phytochemicals and food factors in each food in every meal, every day. Variety within the food groups, as well as among the food groups, also gives tremendous power to your diet. This diet is 46 percent carbohydrates, 31 percent fats and 23 percent protein.

Snack Time!

In addition to the three meals per day listed in the Power-Immunity Diet meal plan, you can have two daily snacks. These can be around exercise (one before and one after) or if you are not working out, then one in the morning and one in the afternoon.

Optimally you will place the pre- and postworkout snacks exactly before and after you exercise, whenever that is during the day. However, if you exercise immediately after a meal or within 30 minutes of your next meal, move the pre- and/or postworkout snacks to another time during the day when a snack will break up a period of longer than three hours between meals.

SNACK 1:

- 1 cup plain low-fat yogurt (not Greek)
- ½ cup fresh berries, halved
- 1 tbsp flaxseed, ground (or 1½ tbsp flaxseed meal)
- ½ ounce (about 1 tbsp) slivered or sliced almonds

SNACK 2:

Smoothie — blend together:
- 1 cup nonfat milk
- ½ fresh banana (frozen is best)
- ½ cup frozen berries
- ½ scoop (10 grams) whey protein isolate (look for one with no additives)

SNACK 3:

- One serving of Almond Butter Whey Cookies (p. 270)

SWEET TREATS

Once per week, you can treat yourself with **one serving** of only one of these snacks:

Preworkout
- Mini Chocolate Soufflés (p. 269)

Postworkout
- Peppermint Protein Ice Cream (p. 273)
- Chocolate Power Pudding (p. 274)

For more tips on treats, see p. 183.

YOUR POWER-IMMUNITY CHEAT SHEET

Simple tips to help you choose the best fuel for your body!

- Emphasize organic, pasture-fed and local products (especially when purchasing animal products) whenever possible.

- Canned tuna should be sustainably-fished catch from troll-caught albacore tuna. It should be minimally processed with at least 7 g of fat per 2 oz serving to ensure a high DHA content. Jig-caught young fish are virtually mercury free. Go to www.tunatuna.com for great products. (We have no financial association with this brand.)

- Include a variety of teas: green, black, oolong, herbal. They all have wonderful antioxidant properties.

- If you like spicy foods, definitely add fresh peppers and pepper spices. These are great metabolic boosters.

- We strongly suggest that you add a daily multivitamin-mineral supplement and a daily probiotic supplement (for more about this topic see the supplements section of this book, p. 190).

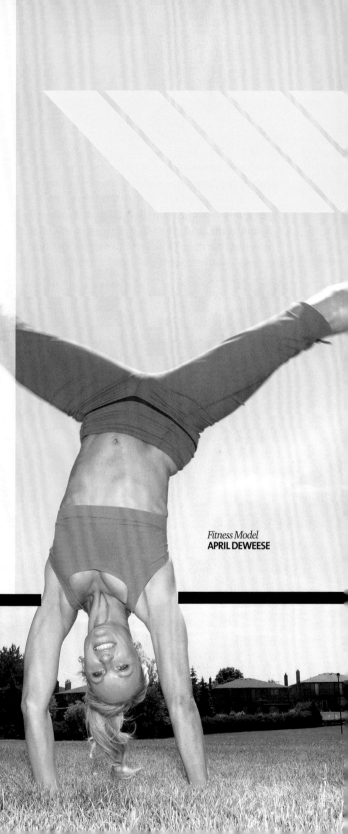

Fitness Model
APRIL DEWEESE

POWER-IMMUNITY DIET MEAL PLAN

BEFORE YOU BEGIN:

Follow this meal plan twice for the 28-day plan.

If the variety of the plan has you feeling overwhelmed, you can choose a few of your favorites and then repeat them. You can swap one breakfast for another, or one lunch for another, or one dinner for another. But don't swap dinner for lunch, or breakfast for dinner and so on.

If absolutely necessary, you can also switch the order of meals within one day, but ideally you should not.

*

* You will be having the Simple Dressing on an almost daily basis. For recipe, see p. 82.

** This fish dish can be substituted with the Grilled Raspberry Salmon on p. 266.

DAY 1

BREAKFAST
Omelette: In a nonstick pan, cook 1 egg (organic, free roaming hens) + 1 tbsp chopped leeks + 2 tbsp diced tomato; 1 slice oat bran toast sprinkled with cinnamon; grape juice spritzer: ⅓ cup concord grape juice with sparkling water; 2 cups water; coffee/tea

LUNCH
Large salad: 2 cups mixed greens + ½ cup sliced cucumber + ¼ cup sliced mushrooms + ¼ cup diced red pepper + ⅓ cup diced avocado + 2 oz grilled chicken, sliced + Simple Dressing*; 4–6 (½ oz) low-fat whole wheat crackers or crispbreads; apple; 2 cups water; tea/other non-caloric beverage

DINNER
Grilled fish:** 3 oz grilled fish of your choice, seasoned with 1 tsp EVOO (extra-virgin olive oil) + ½ tbsp lemon juice, sea salt, pepper; 12 asparagus spears grilled with 1 tsp EVOO + crushed garlic; **Large salad:** 1 cup mixed greens + 1 cup raw spinach + ½ cup mung bean sprouts + 3 cherry tomatoes + 1 tbsp chopped Italian parsley + 1 tbsp toasted sliced almonds + Simple Dressing*; ⅓ cup cooked quinoa; 2 cups water; tea/other non-caloric beverage

DAY 2

BREAKFAST
Egg tortilla: In a nonstick pan, lightly sauté 1 tbsp minced shallots + 2 tbsp shredded zucchini + 1 tbsp chopped red pepper + 1 egg, slightly beaten. Add egg mixture and 2 tbsp salsa to a 6-inch whole wheat tortilla; Pomegranate juice spritzer: ⅓ cup pomegranate juice with sparkling water and fresh lime juice; 2 cups water; coffee/tea

LUNCH
Chicken veggie stir-fry (see note, p. 82): Sauté 2 oz chicken breast strips + 3 cups sliced mixed vegetables + 1½ tsp peanut oil + 2 tsp minced garlic + ½ tsp sesame seeds + 1 tbsp low-sodium soy sauce (add at end of cooking); ⅔ cup brown rice; 1 orange; 2 cups water; tea/other non-caloric beverage

DINNER
Scallops with beets and greens: Lightly sauté 3 oz sea scallops + 1½ tsp olive oil + ½ tbsp minced garlic + 2 tbsp chopped leeks; steam 2 cups Swiss chard + 1 cup cubed golden beets and toss with ½ tsp olive oil + herbs; ⅓ cup polenta; **Small salad:** 1 cup mixed greens + sliced radishes + 1 tbsp chopped parsley + 1 tbsp chopped basil + 1 small tomato, sliced + Simple Dressing*; 2 cups water; tea/other non-caloric beverage

DAY 3

BREAKFAST
Immunity-Boosting Muesli (p. 213); 2 cups water; coffee/tea

LUNCH
Large tuna salad: 2 cups mixed greens + ½ cup steamed green string beans + 3 red onion slices + 3 cherry tomatoes + 2 oz fresh grilled or canned tuna (see note, p. 81) + Simple Dressing*; 4–6 (½ oz) low-fat whole wheat crackers or crispbreads; 1 cup mixed berries; 2 cups water; tea/other non-caloric beverage

DINNER
Halibut stir-fry: Sauté ½ cup mushrooms + raw garlic + 2 tbsp onions + 1 stalk chopped celery + 1 cup broccoli florets + 3 oz sliced halibut fillet seasoned with low-sodium soy sauce, ginger, and 1 tsp canola oil in nonstick wok or pan; ⅓ cup cooked quinoa; **Large salad:** 1 cup shredded red and green cabbage + 1 cup shredded bok choy + ½ tsp toasted sesame seeds + Simple Dressing*; 2 cups water; tea/other non-caloric beverage

DAY 4

BREAKFAST
½ cup mashed soft tofu mixed with 2 tbsp shredded carrot + 2 tbsp chopped cucumber + 2 tbsp shredded broccoli stalk or celery + 1 tbsp chopped parsley + 1 tsp chopped fresh dill + salt and pepper to taste; 1 slice oat bran toast sprinkled with cinnamon; ¾ cup fresh pineapple; 2 cups water; coffee/tea

LUNCH
EAT OUT! Vietnamese restaurant: Order sweet and sour fish stew + 2 fresh vegetable salad rolls; orange spritzer: ½ cup orange juice with sparkling water; 2 cups water; tea/other non-caloric beverage

DINNER
Lamb chops and greens: 3 oz grilled lamb chops sprinkled with fresh lemon juice + 1 cup roasted Brussels sprouts (tossed in ½ tsp EVOO); 1 cup winter squash or ½ cup yam sprinkled with 1 tbsp pomegranate seeds; **Large salad:** 2 cups mixed greens + ½ cup sliced cucumber + ¼ cup sliced mushrooms + ¼ cup diced red pepper + 1 tbsp diced avocado + Simple Dressing*; 2 cups water; tea/other non-caloric beverage

DAY 5

BREAKFAST
Egg lettuce rolls: 2 large romaine lettuce leaves + 1 hard-boiled egg, diced + 1 tbsp shredded carrot + 1 tbsp diced celery + 1 tbsp chopped scallions, mixed with 1 tsp low-fat mayonnaise + ½ tsp mustard. Place ½ egg mixture onto each lettuce leaf and roll up; ½ grapefruit; 2 cups water; coffee/tea

LUNCH
Chicken sandwich: 2 oz grilled chicken breast, sliced or deli chicken + baby spinach leaves, basil leaves and tomato slices + 3 avocado slices + mustard on 2 slices of whole-grain bread; **Small salad:** mixed greens + Simple Dressing*; apple; 2 cups water; tea/other non-caloric beverage

DINNER
Steak with olive tapenade and cucumber: 3 oz grilled tenderloin + ½ cup sautéed mushrooms and onions; 1½ cups chard + 1 tsp EVOO and garlic; 1 tbsp olive tapenade + ½ cup sliced cucumber (spread tapenade on cucumber slices); 1 cup winter squash or ½ cup yam sprinkled with 1 tbsp pomegranate seeds; **Large salad:** 1½ cups mixed greens + sliced mixed veggies + Simple Dressing*; 2 cups water; tea/other non-caloric beverage

DAY 6

BREAKFAST
1 egg prepared any way; 1 slice whole-grain toast topped with 1–2 tbsp plain yogurt and sliced tomato and cucumber; ½ fresh grapefruit; 2 cups water; coffee/tea

LUNCH
Tuna salad sandwich: 2 oz tuna + 1 dill pickle, finely chopped + ¼ tsp minced ginger + ¼ tsp curry powder + 1 tsp reduced-fat mayonnaise + lettuce leaves on 2 slices oat bran bread; Broccoli and cauliflower florets on the side dipped in ¼ cup plain yogurt with fresh dill, minced chives, salt and pepper; 1 cup cherries; 2 cups water; tea/other non-caloric beverage

DINNER
No-Butter Chicken (p. 245); Large salad: 2 cups mixed greens + ½ cup steamed green string beans + 3 red onion slices + 3 cherry tomatoes + Simple Dressing*; 2 cups water; tea/other non-caloric beverage

DAY 7

BREAKFAST
Wonder Woman Yogurt Parfait (p. 277); 2 cups water; coffee/tea

LUNCH
Salmon salad: 2 oz wild grilled or canned salmon + 2 cups mixed greens + 1 stalk celery, chopped + ½ cup broccoli florets + 1 tbsp chopped fresh dill + 1 tbsp toasted sunflower seeds + Simple Dressing*; 4–6 (½ oz) low-fat whole wheat crackers or crispbreads; 1 orange; 2 cups water; tea/other non-caloric beverage

DINNER
Bison burger with layered salad: 3 oz broiled bison burger + baby spinach leaves, tomato, onion, mustard and 2 tsp catsup on 1 whole-grain slider bun; 12 asparagus spears tossed with garlic and grilled; layer together 1 medium tomato, sliced + fresh basil leaves + drizzle with ½ tsp EVOO + 1 tsp balsamic vinegar; 2 cups water; tea/other non-caloric beverage

THE POWER-IMMUNITY DIET MEAL PLAN

SIMPLE DRESSING

You will be eating a large salad almost every day topped with this fat-blasting vinaigrette mix.

1 tbsp extra virgin olive oil

2 tsp red wine vinegar

Sea salt and pepper, to taste

Mix all ingredients in a small bowl or mason jar. Pour over salad. Makes 1 serving. You can make a larger batch and measure out one 1½-tbsp serving per salad.

Nutrients per serving:
Calories: 126, Total Fat: 14 g,
Saturated fat: 2 g, Trans Fat: 0 g,
Cholesterol: 0 mg, Sodium: 8.5 mg,
Total Carbohydrates: 0 g,
Dietary Fiber: 0 g, Sugars: 0 g,
Protein: 0 g, Iron: 0 mg

STIR-FRY TIP

When a stir-fry recipe calls for mixed vegetables, feel free to use any combination of the following abs-firming picks: broccoli, onions, carrots, zucchini, red pepper, red cabbage, mushrooms, snow peas, water chestnuts and bean sprouts.

DAY 8

BREAKFAST
Egg tortilla: In a nonstick pan, lightly sauté 1 tbsp minced shallots + 2 tbsp shredded zucchini + 1 tbsp chopped red pepper + 1 egg, slightly beaten. Add egg mixture and 2 tbsp salsa to a 6-inch whole-wheat tortilla; Pomegranate juice spritzer: ⅓ cup pomegranate juice with sparkling water and fresh lime; 2 cups water; coffee/tea

LUNCH
Chicken & Fire-Roasted Corn Lettuce Wraps (p. 230); fresh fruit cup; 2 cups water, tea/other non-caloric beverage

DINNER
Scallops (or other seafood) with beets and greens: Lightly sauté 3 oz sea scallops + 1½ tsp olive oil + ⅓ tbsp minced garlic + 2 tbsp chopped leeks; steam 2 cups Swiss chard + 1 cup cubed golden or red beets + toss with ½ tsp olive oil and herbs; ⅓ cup polenta sprinkled with 1 tbsp Parmesan cheese and chopped chives; **Small salad:** 1 cup mixed greens + sliced radishes + 1 tbsp chopped parsley + 1 small tomato, sliced + Simple Dressing*; 2 cups water; tea/other non-caloric beverage

DAY 9

BREAKFAST
Omelette: In a nonstick pan, cook 1 egg + 1 tbsp chopped green pepper and 1 tbsp chopped cilantro + 2 tbsp salsa; 1 slice oat bran toast; Grape juice spritzer: ⅓ cup concord grape juice with sparkling water; 2 cups water; coffee/tea

LUNCH
Large tuna salad: 2 oz fresh grilled or canned tuna (see note, p. 81) + 2 cups mixed greens + ½ cup steamed green string beans + 3 red onion slices + 3 cherry tomatoes + Simple Dressing*; 4–6 (½ oz) low-fat whole-wheat crackers or crisp-breads; 1 cup mixed berries; 2 cups water; tea/other non-caloric beverage

DINNER
Spaghetti with meatballs: ½ cup cooked Barilla Plus pasta (high protein/fiber/omega-3) + 3 oz dark turkey meatballs + ¼ cup mushrooms + ½ cup zucchini + garlic + ½ tsp olive oil + ½ cup organic, canned, chopped tomatoes in liquid or sauce + topped with 1 tbsp grated Parmesan cheese (optional); **Large salad:** 2 cups mixed greens + 6 sliced radishes + 1 tbsp fresh chopped parsley + 1 tbsp chopped red pepper + Simple Dressing*; 2 cups water; tea/other non-caloric beverage

DAY 10

BREAKFAST
½ cup mashed soft tofu mixed with 2 tbsp shredded carrot + 2 tbsp chopped cucumber + 2 tbsp shredded broccoli stalk or celery + 1 tbsp chopped parsley + 1 tsp chopped fresh dill, salt and pepper to taste; 1 slice oat bran toast sprinkled with cinnamon; ¾ cup fresh pineapple; 2 cups water; coffee/tea

LUNCH
EAT OUT! Vietnamese restaurant: Order sweet and sour fish stew + 2 fresh vegetable salad rolls; fresh fruit cup; cups water; tea/other non-caloric beverage

DINNER
Lamb chops and greens: 3 oz grilled lamb chops + 1 cup roasted Brussels sprouts (tossed in ½ tsp EVOO); 1 cup winter squash or ½ cup yam sprinkled with 1 tbsp pomegranate seeds; **Large salad:** 2 cups mixed greens + ½ cup sliced cucumber + ¼ cup sliced mushrooms + ¼ cup diced red pepper + 1 tbsp diced avocado + Simple Dressing*; 2 cups water; tea/other non-caloric beverage

DAY 11

BREAKFAST
Egg foo young omelette:
In a nonstick pan, cook
1 egg + 2 tbsp chopped
scallions + ¼ cup mung
bean sprouts + ¼ cup
sliced mushrooms + ⅓ cup
brown rice + ½ tsp low-
sodium soy sauce; ¾ cup
fresh pineapple; 2 cups
water; coffee/tea

LUNCH
Tuna salad sandwich: 2 oz
tuna (see note, p. 81) +
1 dill pickle, finely chopped
+ ¼ tsp minced ginger +
¼ tsp curry powder + 1 tsp
reduced-fat mayonnaise +
lettuce leaves on 2 slices
oat bran bread; broccoli
and cauliflower florets on
the side dipped in ¼ cup
plain yogurt with fresh dill,
minced chives, salt and
pepper; 1 cup cherries;
2 cups water; tea/other
non-caloric beverage

DINNER
Turkey with veggies:
3 oz roast turkey (dark
meat) + 1 cup roasted
Brussels sprouts, tossed
in ½ tsp EVOO + ½ cup
roasted red pepper, sliced;
½ cup baked yam or 1 cup
winter squash seasoned
with a cinnamon and
nutmeg; Large salad:
1 cup mixed greens + 1 cup
raw spinach + ½ cup mung
bean sprouts + 3 cherry
tomatoes + 1 tbsp chopped
Italian parsley + Simple
Dressing*; 2 cups water;
tea/other non-caloric
beverage

DAY 12

BREAKFAST
1 cup Kashi 7 Whole Grain
Puffs + 1 tbsp wheat bran
+ 1 tsp wheat germ +
½ cup plain nonfat Greek
yogurt + 2 tbsp dried fruit
+ cinnamon; 2 cups water;
coffee/tea

LUNCH
EAT OUT! Subway: Order
any 6-inch "Fresh Fit"
sub on the menu (limit
condiments to vinegar,
salt and pepper) OR order
any "Fresh Fit for Kids"
sub + apple slices; 2 cups
water; Tea/other non-
caloric beverage OR Tuna
salad sandwich: 2 oz tuna
(see note, p. 81) + 1 dill
pickle, finely chopped +
¼ tsp minced ginger + ¼
tsp curry powder + 1 tsp
reduced-fat mayonnaise +
lettuce leaves on 2 slices
oat bran bread; broccoli
and cauliflower florets on
the side dipped in ¼ cup
plain yogurt with fresh dill,
minced chives, salt and
pepper; 1 cup cherries;
2 cups water; tea/other
non-caloric beverage

DINNER
Seared Ahi Tuna on Kale
Salad (p. 257); ⅓ cup
brown rice; 2 cups water;
tea/other non-caloric
beverage

DAY 13

BREAKFAST
1 egg, prepared any way;
1 slice whole-grain toast
topped with 1–2 tbsp plain
yogurt and sliced tomato
and cucumber; ½ fresh
grapefruit; 2 cups water;
coffee/tea

LUNCH
Chicken sandwich: 2 oz
grilled chicken breast,
sliced or deli chicken +
lettuce leaves and tomato
slices + 3 avocado slices +
mustard on 2 slices whole-
grain bread; Large salad:
mixed greens + Simple
Dressing*; apple; 2 cups
water; tea/other non-
caloric beverage

DINNER
EAT OUT! Japanese
restaurant: Order 6 pieces
of sushi (with brown
rice) + seaweed salad +
cucumber sunomono (a
small vinegar-based salad)
+ miso soup; 2 cups water;
tea/other non-caloric
beverage

DAY 14

BREAKFAST
½ cup cooked oatmeal +
1 tbsp wheat bran +
1 tsp wheat germ + ½ cup
plain nonfat Greek yogurt;
2 tbsp dried fruit; 2 cups
water; coffee/tea

LUNCH
Raspberry Salmon Salad:
2 oz wild grilled or canned
salmon + 2 cups mixed
greens + 1 stalk celery,
chopped + 2 tbsp
pomegranate seeds +
2 tbsp toasted walnut
pieces + 1 tbsp raspberry
vinegar and 1 tsp EVOO,
freshly ground salt and
pepper; 4–6 (½ oz) low-fat
whole wheat crackers or
crispbreads; orange;
2 cups water; tea/other
non-caloric beverage

DINNER
Roasted chicken with
Kale Chips: 3 oz roasted
chicken + 2 cups Kale Chips
(p. 222); ½ cup steamed
parsnips or baked potato
sprinkled with 1 tbsp
Parmesan cheese; Large
salad: 2 cups mixed greens
+ ½ cup steamed green
string beans + 3 red onion
rings + 3 cherry tomatoes
+ Simple Dressing*; 2 cups
water; tea/other non-
caloric beverage

Your Yoga Workout

Excessive stress, or perhaps more precisely, our reaction to stressors, can wreak havoc on our immune system. In fact, stress can bring about a downward spiral, where stress causes a lowered immune system, and then illness acts as a stressor to lower the immune system further still.

You've probably heard of psychosomatic illness. Often we think of this as being an illness that's "all in our head" – in other words, an imagined illness. But a psychosomatic illness is a real illness caused by factors in our head – commonly stress. We cannot avoid stressors in our lives, but we can do our best to react to those stressors in as healthy a way as possible. We can do that by avoiding drugs and excessive alco-

hol, by eating healthfully, exercising regularly (and vigorously) and by learning to relax. For more stress-fighting advice, see the "Healthy Body, Healthy Mind" section of this book, p. 118.

Yoga is a great way to combine exercise and relaxation. Although we don't suggest yoga should take the place of cardio and weight training, it can certainly act as a great addition to any physical fitness program. The following poses are not especially challenging; they are relaxation poses. Make sure to breathe very deeply, slowly and evenly throughout these poses. Hold each pose for at least 30 seconds but as long as you like. While you are holding the pose, make sure you do not allow your posture to slip.

1// *Easy Pose*

SET-UP/ Sit on the floor, posture erect and legs straight in front.

ACTION/ This pose may remind you of your kindergarten days. Fold your legs one at a time, bringing them close to your body as you do so, and tucking each foot under the opposite leg's calf. Rest your hands on your knees.

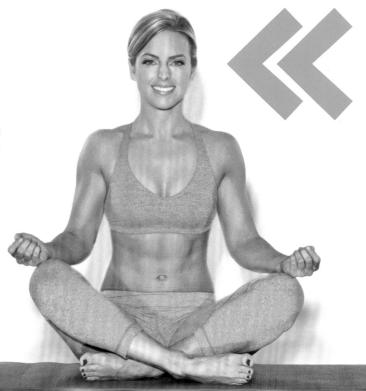

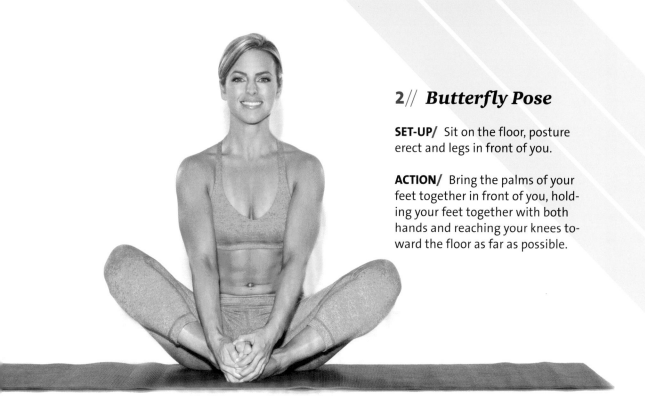

2// *Butterfly Pose*

SET-UP/ Sit on the floor, posture erect and legs in front of you.

ACTION/ Bring the palms of your feet together in front of you, holding your feet together with both hands and reaching your knees toward the floor as far as possible.

3// *Child's Pose*

SET-UP/ Kneel on the floor, your toes touching but knees about hip-width apart.

ACTION/ Exhaling, bring your torso down to rest on your thighs. Bring your arms back along your sides, palms facing up. Consciously widen your back and elongate your neck, feeling the weight of your shoulders widen your upper back.

4// *Knees-to-Chest Pose*

SET-UP/ Lie on your back on a mat or rug.

ACTION/ Bring your knees up to your chest, bending your legs. Clasp your hands together around your shins.

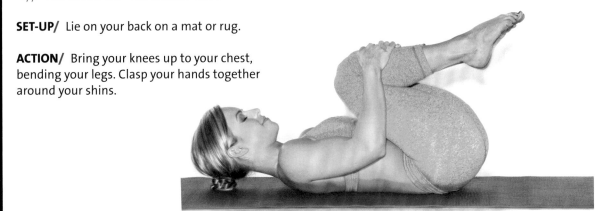

5// *Reclined Spinal Twist*

SET-UP/ Lie on your back on a mat or rug, legs straight and in line with your body.

ACTION/ Leaving one leg straight, bring one knee up in a twisting motion to its opposite side, touching the floor, exactly perpendicular to your body (and straight leg). Your arms will be lying straight out directly from the body, parallel to the thigh of the bent leg. If needed, you can use one hand to help your knee stay down, as shown. Turn your head to face the direction opposite your bent knee.

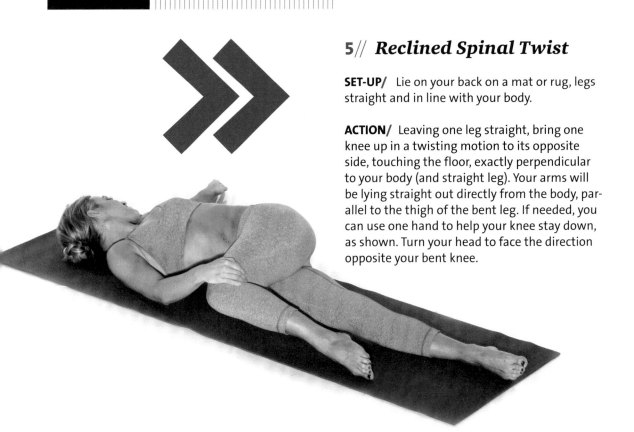

6// *Corpse Pose*

SET-UP/ Lie on your back on a mat or rug, legs fully extended.

ACTION/ Use your hands to tilt the back of your head slightly away from your neck and then extend your arms beside your body, hands about six to eight inches from your hips, palms facing the ceiling. Allow your feet to fall apart in a relaxed manner, evenly on both sides.

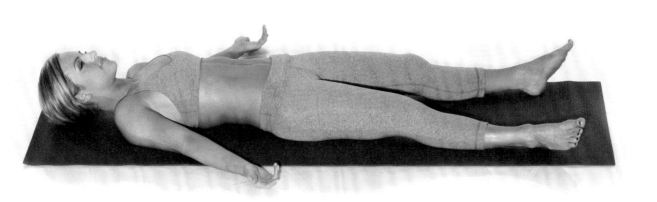

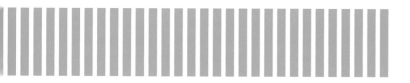

The **Oxygen Diet Solution** *Success* Story

ONCE SHE FOUND HER GROOVE, DENYSE RAYNOR NEVER LOOKED BACK. SHE LOST 65 POUNDS!

"I am healthy from the inside out!"

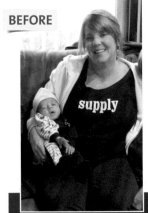

BEFORE

BEFORE: 200 lb

NOW: 135 lb

AGE: 44

HEIGHT: 5'5"

LOCATION: Bel Air, MD

OCCUPATION: Software sales executive

FAVORITE EXERCISE:
Lying leg curl

Weighing in at 200 pounds following the birth of her fifth child, Denyse Raynor met with a personal trainer. Admiring a fitness competitor nearby, Denyse pointed at the fit woman and said, "I want to do what that girl's doing!" And she was off.

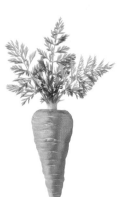

Fitness Inspiration

When she was 16, Denyse's grandfather ("Pop-Pop" to Denyse) was diagnosed with colon cancer. Determined to outlive his prognosis, he began exercising daily and eating nutrient-rich, chemical-free whole foods – with great success. Twenty years later, he explained to Denyse that what was important was how you looked on the *inside*. So when she started reading nutrition articles in *Oxygen*, things clicked. Less than a year after she'd set out on her mission, Denyse had ditched 65 pounds, reshaped her body and competed in her first figure show, going shoulder-to-shoulder, at age 41, with women 20 years younger.

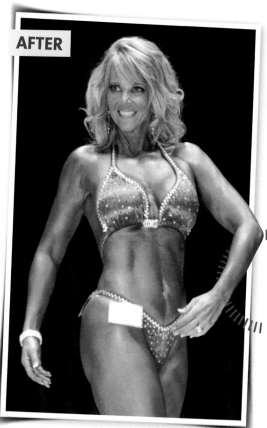

AFTER

> *"Many people face obstacles. We make a decision to overcome them, or let them overcome us."*

Energizer Mommy

Over time, Denyse's gym attire went from sweats, to yoga pants, to shorts and fitted tops. "My stomach has been the hardest thing for me to lose after having the kids," she says. Denyse trains abs once a week, and it shows. "I'm much more confident now!" she says.

Pop-Pop's Omelette

Denyse starts her mornings with a clean egg dish that's been passed down to her from her grandfather.

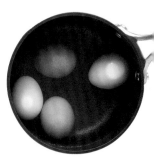

TRY IT:

1. Mix together 1 whole egg, 5 egg whites, a handful of fresh spinach and pour into a nonstick pan.

2. When firm, flip over. Spread ⅓ cup low-fat cottage cheese on top.

3. Flip one side over and slide omelette onto a plate.

Mood Boosters

"I am definitely an emotional eater," says Denyse, so when she's feeling down, she chooses one of these different paths: Listening to upbeat music; going out for coffee with a girlfriend; calling a supportive friend.

Success Prep

Denyse had to conquer the "cardio queen" mindset and focus on weights. To stay motivated, she filed inspirational materials – recipes, workouts and photos of her favorite fitness models – in a "fitness folder" she kept at work. She tracked short- and long-term goals on a calendar.

Cardio Faves

When she isn't lifting weights in the gym, Denyse still loves to burn calories with cardio. Her favorite aerobic exercises include:

- Using the elliptical machine

- Using the StepMill

- Walking stairs (alternating every step with every other step)

- Treadmill incline walk

- Treadmill interval jog

- Aerobics classes

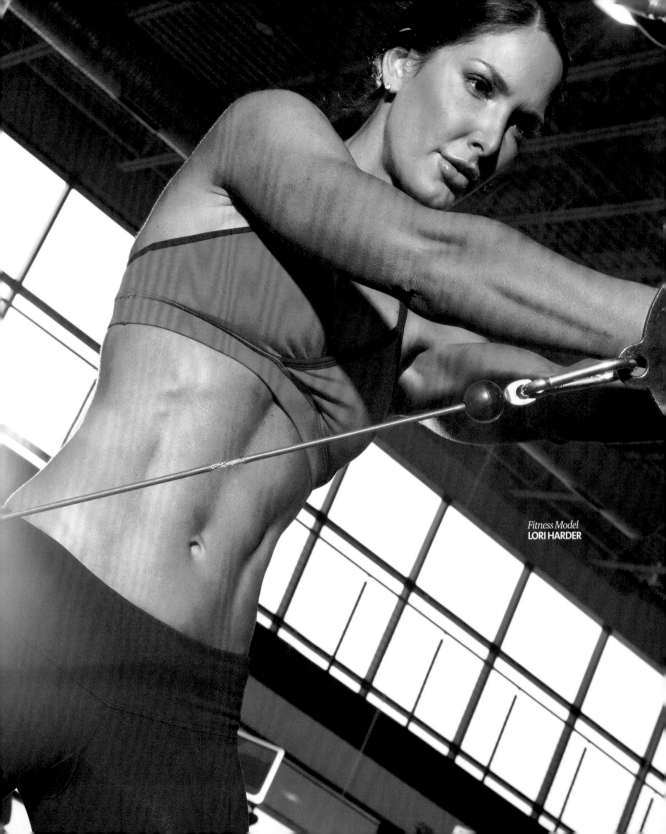

Fitness Model
LORI HARDER

Muscle-Building Diet

Create a sexy, toned body

Eye-popping abs, sleek and sexy arms, glorious glutes …
Just flipping through a fitness magazine or even the pages
of this book can make some women burn with a bitter mix
of envy and frustration. This is usually because they think
owning a body like that is only a pipe dream – but it's not!
Achieving the body of your dreams is possible, no matter
what your weight and shape are now. In fact, plenty of top
fitness models, including Tosca Reno, Tiffani Bachus, Chady
Dunmore and Rita Catolino, were once overweight. And
during their transformations, they all came to the realization that they could quite literally design and build their
own bodies to look exactly the way they wanted them to.
So remember, with hard work and dedication, you too can
achieve that same wonderful realization.

That lean, toned look we love so much comes from two sources – having low body fat and building muscle. Many women still mistakenly think they will bulk up like Schwarzenegger if they lift weights, but this is simply not true. The reality is that to get bodies like those of the women you see in *Oxygen* magazine and throughout this book, you will need to lift weights, and quite heavy weights at that.

But exercise is only part of the equation. Muscle is stressed in the gym but built when you are at rest, and the bricks and mortar of muscle is food. Many diets do not support muscle building because they don't offer enough food, don't offer enough of specific nutrients, or both.

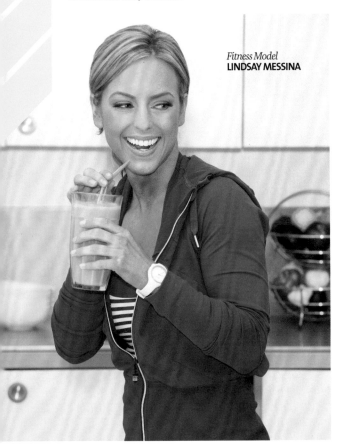

Fitness Model
LINDSAY MESSINA

Protein is the obvious, even stereotypical, muscle-building nutrient, and indeed it is important, but you cannot build muscle on protein alone. Without carbohydrates, we would not be able to even perform our workouts let alone build muscle from them. Carbohydrates break down into simple sugars, which our entire body (including our brain) uses for instant energy. Whatever is not used immediately is converted to muscle glycogen, which is the energy we use to move our muscles, so you can see how a lack of carbohydrates might affect your performance in the gym. Consuming carbohydrates after training also puts our body in an anabolic (muscle-building) state, so make sure to add some carbs to that post-workout shake!

With the widespread popularity of low-carb diets such as *The Dukan Diet* and *The 17-Day Diet*, carbs have recently become a four-letter word. The same was said of fats in the 1990s. "Fat makes you fat!" was a common refrain, and chemical-laden low-fat (but often high-calorie) products began sprouting up on shelves like weeds. It turns out, however, that thinking was quite far from the truth. Healthy fats actually help keep you lean (they take longer to digest so you end up feeling full longer), they help you build muscle and they help your body absorb essential vitamins.

This doesn't mean you should start chowing down on sausages, cream cheese and butter. Saturated fats, trans fats and any processed foods aid weight gain and poor health. The fats you should be eating are monounsaturated and polyunsaturated. Mono fats include olive oil, almonds, seeds, avocados and natural nut butters. Poly fats are made up of omega-3 and omega-6 fatty acids and are found in soybean and canola oils, walnuts, tuna, wild salmon and other coldwater fish.

To build healthy muscle, you need a balance of protein with good carbs and healthy fats – which this diet provides.

Your Muscle-Building Diet Meal Plan

The following muscle-building diet is made up of 40 percent carbohydrates, 30 percent protein and 30 percent fat, and it contains enough calories to build up that sexy muscle while keeping you lean.

Snack Time!

In addition to the three meals per day listed in the Muscle-Building Diet meal plan, you can have two daily snacks. These can be around exercise (one before and one after) or if you are not working out, then one in the morning and one in the afternoon.

Optimally you will place the pre- and postworkout snacks exactly before and after you exercise, whenever that is during the day. However, if you exercise immediately after a meal or within 30 minutes of your next meal, move the pre- and/or postworkout snacks to another time during the day when a snack will break up a period of longer than three hours between meals.

SNACK 1:
- 1 cup plain nonfat Greek yogurt
- ½ cup fresh berries, halved
- ½ ounce (about 1 tbsp) slivered or sliced almonds

SNACK 2
Smoothie – blend together:
- 1 cup nonfat milk
- ½ banana (frozen is best)
- ½ cup frozen berries
- 1 scoop (20 grams) whey protein isolate (look for one with no additives)

SNACK 3 (POSTWORKOUT ONLY)
- Spelt Flatbread With Yogurt Dip (see p. 221)

SNACK 4
- One serving of Almond Butter Whey Cookies (p. 270)

SWEET TREATS
Once per week, you can treat yourself with **one serving** of only one of these snacks:

Preworkout
- Mini Chocolate Soufflés (p. 269)

Postworkout
- Peppermint Protein Ice Cream (p. 273)
- Chocolate Power Pudding (p. 274)

For more tips on treats, see p. 183.

MUSCLE-BUILDING DIET MEAL PLAN

BEFORE YOU BEGIN:

Follow this meal plan twice for the 28-day plan.

If the variety of the plan has you feeling overwhelmed, you can choose a few of your favorites and then repeat them. You can swap one breakfast for another, or one lunch for another, or one dinner for another. But don't swap dinner for lunch, or breakfast for dinner and so on.

If absolutely necessary, you can also switch the order of meals within one day, but ideally you should not.

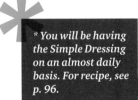

You will be having the Simple Dressing on an almost daily basis. For recipe, see p. 96.

DAY 1

BREAKFAST
Omelette: In a nonstick pan, cook 1 egg + 1 tbsp chopped onions or scallions + 1 tbsp diced tomato; 1 slice whole-grain toast, ½ cup orange juice; 2 cups water; coffee/tea

LUNCH
Large salad: 2 cups mixed greens + ½ cup sliced cucumber + ¼ cup sliced mushrooms + ¼ cup diced red pepper + ⅓ cup avocado; diced + 4 oz sliced grilled chicken + Simple Dressing*; 4–6 (½ oz) low-fat whole wheat crackers or crispbreads; 2 cups water; tea/other non-caloric beverage

DINNER
Grilled salmon: 4 oz grilled wild salmon, seasoned with 1 tsp EVOO (extra-virgin olive oil) + ½ tbsp lemon juice, sea salt, pepper; 12 asparagus spears tossed with 1 tsp EVOO + crushed garlic and grilled; Large salad: 1 cup mixed greens + 1 cup raw spinach + ½ cup mung bean sprouts + 3 cherry tomatoes + 1 tbsp chopped Italian parsley + 1 tbsp toasted sliced almonds + Simple Dressing*, ½ cup cooked quinoa, 2 cups water, tea/other non-caloric beverage

DAY 2

BREAKFAST
Egg tortilla: In a nonstick pan, lightly sauté: 1 tbsp minced shallots + 2 tbsp shredded zucchini + 1 tbsp chopped red pepper + 1 egg, slightly beaten. Add egg mixture and 2 tbsp salsa to 1 (6-inch) whole-wheat tortilla; ½ cup pineapple juice; 2 cups water; coffee/tea

LUNCH
Chicken veggie stir-fry (see tip, p. 96): Sauté 4 oz chicken breast strips + 3 cups sliced mixed vegetables + 1½ tsp peanut oil + 2 tsp minced garlic + ½ tsp sesame seeds + 1 tbsp low-sodium soy sauce (add at end of cooking); ⅔ cup brown rice; 2 cups water; tea/other non-caloric beverage

DINNER
Scallops (or other seafood) with beets and greens: Lightly sauté 4 oz sea scallops + 1½ tsp olive oil + ½ tbsp minced garlic; steam 2 cups Swiss chard + 1 cup cubed golden or red beets + toss with ½ tsp olive oil and herbs; ½ cup polenta; Small salad: 1 cup mixed greens + sliced radishes + 1 tbsp chopped parsley + 1 small tomato, sliced + Simple Dressing*; 2 cups water; tea/other non-caloric beverage

DAY 3

BREAKFAST
Egg foo young omelette: In a nonstick pan, cook 1 egg + 2 tbsp chopped scallions + ¼ cup mung bean sprouts + ¼ cup sliced mushrooms + ⅓ cup brown rice + ½ tsp low-sodium soy sauce; ½ cup orange juice; 2 cups water; coffee/tea

LUNCH
Large tuna salad: 2 cups mixed greens + ½ cup steamed green string beans + 3 red onion slices + 3 cherry tomatoes + 4 oz fresh grilled or canned tuna + Simple Dressing*; 4–6 (½ oz) low-fat whole-wheat crackers or crispbreads; 2 cups water; tea/other non-caloric beverage

DINNER
Roasted chicken with Kale Chips: 4 oz roasted chicken + 2 cups Kale Chips (p. 222); ½ cup steamed parsnips or baked potato; Large salad: 2 cups mixed greens + ½ cup steamed green string beans + 3 red onion slices + 3 cherry tomatoes + 5–6 olives + Simple Dressing*; 2 cups water; tea/other non-caloric beverage

DAY 4

BREAKFAST
½ cup cottage cheese mixed with 2 tbsp shredded carrot + 2 tbsp chopped cucumber + 2 tbsp shredded broccoli stalk or celery + 1 tbsp chopped parsley, salt and pepper to taste; 1 slice whole-grain toast; ½ cup pineapple juice; 2 cups water; coffee/tea

LUNCH
Large tuna salad: 2 cups mixed greens + ½ cup steamed green string beans + 3 red onion slices + 3 cherry tomatoes + 4 oz fresh grilled or canned tuna + Simple Dressing*; 4–6 (½ oz) low-fat whole-wheat crackers or crispbreads; 2 cups water; tea/other non-caloric beverage

DINNER
Roasted chicken with Kale Chips: 4 oz roasted chicken + 2 cups Kale Chips (p. 222); ½ cup steamed parsnips or baked potato; Large salad: 2 cups mixed greens + ½ cup steamed green string beans + 3 red onion slices + 3 cherry tomatoes + 5–6 olives + Simple Dressing*; 2 cups water; tea/other non-caloric beverage

DAY 5

BREAKFAST
Egg lettuce rolls: 2 large iceberg lettuce leaves + 1 hard-boiled egg, diced + 1 tbsp shredded carrot + 1 tbsp diced celery, mixed with 1 tsp low-fat mayonnaise + ½ tsp yellow mustard. Place ½ egg mixture into each lettuce leaf and roll up; ½ grapefruit; 2 cups water; coffee/tea

LUNCH
Chicken sandwich: 4 oz grilled chicken breast, sliced or deli chicken + lettuce leaves and tomato slices + 3 avocado slices + mustard on 2 slices whole-grain bread; Mixed greens salad + Simple Dressing*; 2 cups water; tea/other non-caloric beverage

DINNER
Steak with olive tapenade and cucumber: 4 oz grilled tenderloin + ½ cup sautéed mushrooms and onions; 1½ cups Swiss chard sautéed in 1 tsp EVOO and garlic; 1 tbsp olive tapenade + ½ cup sliced cucumber (spread tapenade on cucumber slices); 1 cup winter squash or ½ cup yam; Large salad: 1½ cups mixed greens + 6 sliced radishes + 1 tbsp fresh chopped parsley + 1 small tomato, sliced + Simple Dressing*; 2 cups water; tea/other non-caloric beverage

DAY 6

BREAKFAST
1 egg prepared any way; 1 slice whole-grain toast topped with 1–2 tbsp plain yogurt and sliced tomato and cucumber; ½ fresh grapefruit; 2 cups water; coffee/tea

LUNCH
Tuna salad sandwich: 4 oz tuna + 1 dill pickle, finely chopped + ¼ tsp minced ginger + ¼ tsp curry powder + 1 tsp low-fat mayonnaise + lettuce leaves on 2 slices whole-grain bread; sliced mixed vegetables on the side; 2 cups water; tea/other non-caloric beverage

DINNER
Roasted chicken with Kale Chips: 4 oz roasted chicken + 2 cups Kale Chips (p. 222); ½ cup steamed parsnips or baked potato; Large salad: 2 cups mixed greens + ½ cup steamed green string beans + 3 red onion slices + 3 cherry tomatoes + Simple Dressing*; 2 cups water; tea/other non-caloric beverage

DAY 7

BREAKFAST
Apple Oatmeal Chocolate Protein Bars (p. 214); Note: When you eat these for breakfast, eliminate 1–2 fat servings from your other meals for the rest of the day; 2 cups water; coffee/tea

LUNCH
Turkey salad: 4 oz sliced turkey breast + 2 cups leafy greens + 1 stalk chopped celery + ½ cup broccoli florets + 1 tbsp toasted sunflower seeds + Simple Dressing*; 4–6 (½ oz) low-fat whole wheat crackers or crispbreads; 2 cups water; tea/other non-caloric beverage

DINNER
Halibut stir-fry: Sauté ½ cup mushrooms + raw garlic + 2 tbsp onions + 1 stalk chopped celery + 1 cup snow peas + 4 oz sliced halibut fillet seasoned with low-sodium soy sauce, ginger, and 1½ tsp canola oil in nonstick wok or pan. Add ½ tsp toasted sesame seeds at end of cooking; ½ cup cooked quinoa; Large salad: 1 cup shredded red and green cabbage + 1 cup shredded bok choy + Simple Dressing*; 2 cups water; tea/other non-caloric beverage

SIMPLE DRESSING

You will be eating a large salad almost every day topped with this fat-blasting vinaigrette mix.

1 tbsp extra virgin olive oil

2 tsp red wine vinegar

Sea salt and pepper, to taste

Mix all ingredients in a small bowl or mason jar. Pour over salad. Makes 1 serving. You can make a larger batch and measure out one 1½ Tbsp serving per salad.

Nutrients per serving:
Calories: 126, Total Fat: 14 g,
Saturated fat: 2 g, Trans Fat: 0 g,
Cholesterol: 0 mg, Sodium: 8.5 mg,
Total Carbohydrates: 0 g,
Dietary Fiber: 0 g, Sugars: 0 g,
Protein: 0 g, Iron: 0 mg

STIR-FRY TIP

When a stir-fry recipe calls for mixed vegetables, feel free to use any combination of the following abs-firming picks: broccoli, onions, carrots, zucchini, red pepper, red cabbage, mushrooms, snow peas, water chestnuts and bean sprouts.

DAY 8

BREAKFAST
Egg tortilla: Lightly sauté in nonstick pan: 1 tbsp minced shallots + 2 tbsp shredded zucchini + 1 tbsp chopped red pepper + 1 egg, slightly beaten. Add egg mixture and 2 tbsp salsa to a 6-inch whole wheat tortilla; ½ cup pineapple juice; 2 cups water; coffee/tea

LUNCH
EAT OUT! Thai restaurant: Order chicken lettuce wraps; fresh fruit cup; 2 cups water; tea/other non-caloric beverage

DINNER
Scallops (or other seafood) with beets and greens: Lightly sauté 4 oz sea scallops + 1½ tsp olive oil + ½ tbsp minced garlic; steam 2 cups Swiss chard + 1 cup cubed golden or red beets + toss with ½ tsp olive oil and herbs; ½ cup polenta; **Small salad:** 1 cup mixed greens + sliced radishes + 1 tbsp chopped parsley + 1 small tomato, sliced + Simple Dressing*; 2 cups water; tea/other non-caloric beverage

DAY 9

BREAKFAST
Omelette: In a nonstick pan, cook 1 egg + 1 tbsp chopped green pepper + 1 tbsp chopped cilantro + 2 tbsp salsa; 1 slice whole-grain toast; ½ cup orange juice; 2 cups water; coffee/tea

LUNCH
Large tuna salad: 4 oz fresh grilled or canned tuna + 2 cups leafy greens + ½ cup steamed green string beans + 3 red onion slices + 3 cherry tomatoes + Simple Dressing*; 4–6 (½ oz) low-fat whole wheat crackers or crispbreads; 2 cups water; tea/other non-caloric beverage

DINNER
Spaghetti with meatballs: ½ cup cooked whole wheat pasta + 4 oz meatballs + ¼ cup mushrooms + ½ cup zucchini + garlic + ½ tsp olive oil + ½ cup organic, canned, chopped tomatoes in liquid or sauce + 1 tbsp grated Parmesan cheese (optional); **Large salad:** 2 cups mixed greens + 6 sliced radishes + 1 tbsp fresh chopped parsley + 1 tbsp chopped red pepper + 5–6 olives + 1 tbsp walnut pieces + Simple Dressing*; 2 cups water; tea/other non-caloric beverage

DAY 10

BREAKFAST
Banana Walnut Protein Pancakes (p. 210); 2 cups water; coffee/tea

LUNCH
EAT OUT! Vietnamese restaurant: Order sweet and sour fish stew + 2 fresh vegetable salad rolls; Fresh fruit cup; 2 cups water; tea/other non-caloric beverage

DINNER
Lamb chops and greens: 4 oz grilled lamb chops + 1 cup roasted Brussels sprouts (tossed in ½ tsp EVOO); 1 cup winter squash or ½ cup yam; **Large salad:** 2 cups mixed greens + ½ cup sliced cucumber + ¼ cup sliced mushrooms + ¼ cup diced red pepper + 1 tbsp diced avocado + 1 tbsp walnut pieces + Simple Dressing*; 2 cups water; tea/other non-caloric beverage

DAY 11

BREAKFAST
Egg foo young omelette:
In a nonstick pan, cook
1 egg + 2 tbsp chopped
scallions + ¼ cup mung
bean sprouts + ¼ cup
sliced mushrooms + ⅓
cup brown rice + ½ tsp low
sodium soy sauce; ½ cup
orange juice; 2 cups water;
coffee/tea

LUNCH
Tuna salad sandwich:
4 oz tuna + 1 dill pickle,
finely chopped + ¼ tsp
minced ginger + ¼ tsp
curry powder + 1 tsp
low-fat mayonnaise +
lettuce leaves on 2 slices
whole-grain bread;
Sliced mixed vegetables
on the side with dip: ¼
cup plain nonfat yogurt
+ ⅛ tsp curry powder +
¼ tsp ketchup + 1 drop
Worcestershire sauce;
2 cups water; tea/other
non-caloric beverage

DINNER
Turkey with veggies: 4 oz
roast turkey (light or dark
meat) + 1 cup roasted
Brussels sprouts (tossed
in 1 tsp EVOO) + ½ cup
roasted red pepper, sliced;
½ cup baked yam or 1 cup
winter squash; Large salad:
1 cup mixed greens +
1 cup raw spinach + ½ cup
mung bean sprouts +
3 cherry tomatoes + 1 tbsp
chopped Italian parsley +
1 tbsp toasted walnut
pieces + Simple Dressing*;
2 cups water; tea/other
non-caloric beverage

DAY 12

BREAKFAST
Omelette: In a nonstick
pan, cook 1 egg + 1 tbsp
chopped green pepper +
1 tbsp chopped cilantro
+ 2 tbsp salsa; 1 slice
whole-grain toast; ½ cup
orange juice; 2 cups water;
coffee/tea

LUNCH
EAT OUT! Subway: Order
any 6-inch "Fresh Fit"
sub on the menu (limit
condiments to vinegar,
salt and pepper) OR order
any "Fresh Fit for Kids" sub
+ apple slices OR Chicken
sandwich: 4 oz grilled
chicken breast, sliced
or deli chicken + lettuce
leaves and tomato slices +
3 avocado slices + mustard
on 2 slices of whole-grain
bread; mixed greens salad
+ Simple Dressing*; 2 cups
water; tea/other non-
caloric beverage

DINNER
Chicken veggie stir-fry
(see tip, p. 96): Sauté 4
oz chicken + 3 cups sliced
mixed vegetables + 2 tsp
peanut oil + 2 tsp minced
garlic + ½ tsp sesame seeds
+ 1 tbsp low-sodium soy
sauce + ½ tsp sesame oil
(add at end of cooking);
⅓ cup brown rice; 2 cups
water; tea/other non-
caloric beverage

DAY 13

BREAKFAST
1 egg prepared any way;
1 slice whole-grain toast
topped with 1–2 tbsp
plain yogurt, sliced tomato
and cucumber; ½ fresh
grapefruit; 2 cups water;
coffee/tea

LUNCH
Chicken sandwich: 4 oz
grilled chicken breast,
sliced or deli chicken +
lettuce leaves and tomato
slices + 3 avocado slices +
mustard on 2 slices whole-
grain bread; mixed greens
salad + Simple Dressing*;
2 cups water; tea/other
non-caloric beverage

DINNER
EAT OUT! Japanese
restaurant: Order 4 pieces
of sushi (with rice) +
4 pieces of sashimi (no
rice) + seaweed salad +
cucumber sunomono (a
small vinegar-based salad)
+ miso soup; 2 cups water;
tea/other non-caloric
beverage

DAY 14

BREAKFAST
½ cup cooked oatmeal;
½ cup Greek plain nonfat
yogurt; 2 tbsp dried fruit;
2 cups water; coffee/tea

LUNCH
Turkey salad: 4 oz sliced
turkey breast + 2 cups
salad green + 1 stalk
chopped celery + ½ cup
broccoli florets + 2 cherry
tomatoes + 1 tbsp toasted
sunflower seeds + Simple
Dressing*; 4–6 (½ oz) low-
fat whole wheat crackers
or crispbreads; 2 cups
water; tea/other non-
caloric beverage

DINNER
Beef Teriyaki (p. 242);
Layer together 1 medium
tomato, sliced + fresh basil
leaves + drizzle with ½ tsp
EVOO + 1 tsp balsamic
vinegar; 5–6 olives; 2 cups
water; tea/other non-
caloric beverage

Workouts

Because your goal is building muscle, your workout schedule will be a little different from the other schedules in this book because it will emphasize weight training. Do three sets of 8–12 reps for each exercise. If you can complete 12 reps easily, increase the weight.

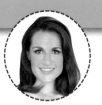
5-Day Plans

 1

MONDAY: 45–75 minutes weight training
TUESDAY: 60 minutes cardio
WEDNESDAY: 45–75 minutes weight training
THURSDAY: 60 minutes cardio
FRIDAY: 45–75 minutes weight training

 2

MONDAY: 45 minutes weight training,
    30 minutes cardio
TUESDAY: 45 minutes weight training,
    30 minutes cardio
WEDNESDAY: 45 minutes weight training,
    30 minutes cardio
THURSDAY: 45 minutes weight training,
    30 minutes cardio
FRIDAY: 45 minutes weight training,
    30 minutes cardio

6-Day Plans

 1

MONDAY: 45–75 minutes weight training
TUESDAY: 45–75 minutes weight training
WEDNESDAY: 60 minutes cardio
THURSDAY: 45–75 minutes weight training
FRIDAY: 45–75 minutes weight training
SATURDAY: 60 minutes cardio

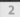 **2**

MONDAY: 45 minutes weight training,
    30 minutes cardio
TUESDAY: 45–75 minutes weight training
WEDNESDAY: 60 minutes cardio
THURSDAY: 45 minutes weight training,
    30 minutes cardio
FRIDAY: 45–75 minutes weight training
SATURDAY: 60 minutes cardio

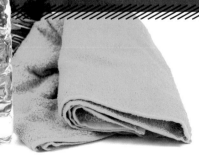

Your Muscle-Building Workout

If you are a beginner to working out with weights, then choose one of the following exercises per body part and do a full-body workout three times per week (see option 1 in the 5-Day Plan section). After a few weeks of working out this way you can begin doing a body part split, training half your body one weight-training day and the other half the next. Dividing into upper and lower body and push and pull exercises are two of the most common splits (i.e., work your upper body one day and your lower body the next, or perform "push" exercises such as bench press and squats one day, and "pull" exercises such as lat pull-downs and hamstring curls the next).

Once you have developed a solid base of muscle you can divide the body up even further, adding more exercises and sets per body part and working each only once per week. Read *Oxygen* for other great exercise selections to vary your routine!

Cardio

Before beginning your training, warm up for five to 10 minutes with some light cardio. This can be anything from jogging to stationary cycling to dancing – whatever gets your blood pumping. Do the exercises in the order shown here (large body parts before smaller ones). Otherwise your small body parts will fatigue more quickly, making you unable to work your big muscles effectively.

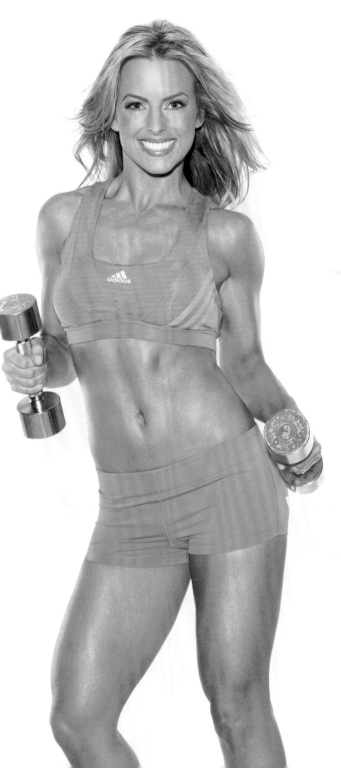

Fitness Model
LINDSAY MESSINA

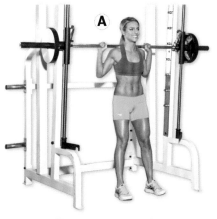

1// *Smith-Machine Squats*

TONES THESE AREAS:
QUADS AND GLUTES

SET UP/ Stand underneath the bar of a Smith machine, bar resting on your shoulders, knees bent, feet shoulder-width apart. Stand up, unhooking the bar from the pins as you do so **[A]**.

ACTION/ Holding the bar across your shoulders, lower down into a squat position, making sure your knees do not travel over your toes **[B]**. Push up to stand again, and repeat.

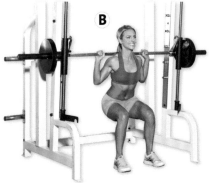

2// *Hamstring Curls*

TONES THESE AREAS:
HAMSTRINGS

SET UP/ Lie facedown on a hamstring curl machine, legs underneath the pads, which are set just above your ankles **[A]**.

ACTION/ Holding the handles for leverage, bring your feet toward your buttocks by bending your knees **[B]**. Slowly lower back down and repeat.

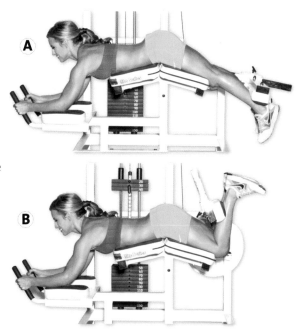

3// *Deadlifts*

TONES THESE AREAS:
GLUTES, LOWER BACK, QUADS

SET UP/ Set a barbell on the floor and stand behind it, legs shoulder-width apart. Squat down and, keeping your back straight, grasp the bar with an overhand grip. Your hands should be about shoulder-width apart **[A]**.

ACTION/ Keeping your back flat and using your legs, lift the bar as you stand up straight, keeping it at arms' length **[B]**. Lower the bar to the floor and continue to repeat, making sure to keep your back flat and to use your legs and glutes to power the movement.

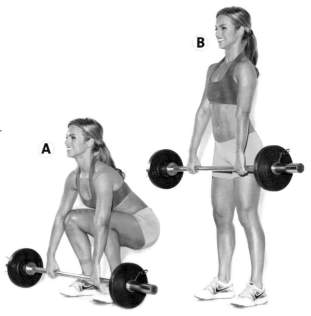

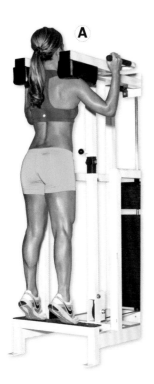

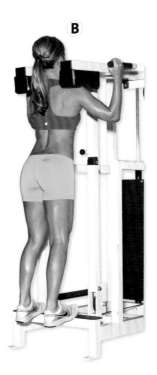

4// *Calf Raises*

TONES THESE AREAS:
CALVES

SET UP/ Stand underneath the shoulder pads of a calf-raise machine, knees slightly bent, toes on the footplate, heels hanging off.

ACTION/ Straighten your legs and come up on your toes as far as you can **[A]**. Lower your heels as far as possible to get a good stretch in your calves **[B]** before lifting them again.

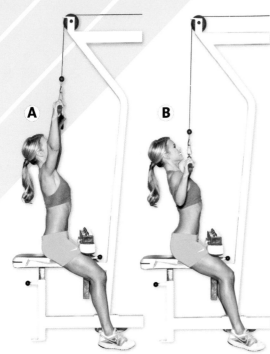

5// *Lat Pulldowns*

TONES THESE AREAS:
BACK, ESPECIALLY LATS

SET UP/ Sit at the lat machine, pad set on your knees. Stand slightly to reach the bar, then sit, holding the bar with arms stretched **[A]**.

ACTION/ Keeping your back flat or arched and staying as upright as possible, pull the weight toward your upper chest using your back muscles **[B]**. Carefully allow the weight back to starting position. Repeat.

6// *Bent-Over Rows*

TONES THESE AREAS:
BACK, ESPECIALLY MID-UPPER BACK,
REAR DELTOIDS (SHOULDERS)

SET UP/ Stand, feet shoulder-width apart, behind a barbell. Bend down and pick up the barbell, using your legs. Bend over, keeping your back flat, holding the weight at arms' length **[A]**.

ACTION/ Lift the barbell to your chest and lower again, keeping your back flat and your eyes forward through the entire movement **[B]**. Repeat.

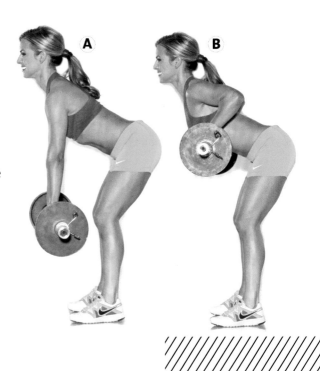

7// *Incline Press*

TONES THESE AREAS:
CHEST, FRONT DELTOIDS (SHOULDERS)

SET UP/ Grasp your selected dumbbells and lie back on a bench inclined to 30 to 40 degrees. Hold the dumbbells at your shoulders **[A]**.

ACTION/ Press the dumbbells straight up and bring in slightly so they meet at the top of the movement **[B]**. Lower back to your shoulders and repeat.

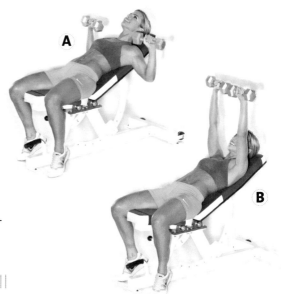

8// *Dumbbell Flyes*

TONES THESE AREAS:
INNER CHEST

SET UP/ Grasp your selected dumbbells and lie back on a bench. Open your arms, elbows slightly bent, holding dumbbells with palms facing the ceiling **[A]**.

ACTION/ Using a hugging motion, bring the dumbbells toward each other, making sure your elbows stay in line with your shoulders **[B]**. Bring back to the open-arm position and repeat.

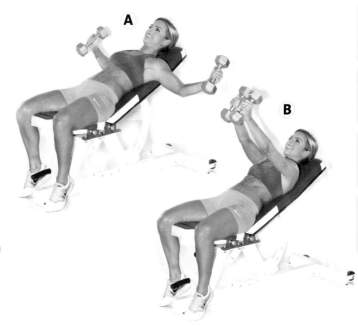

9// *Triceps Dip*

TONES THESE AREAS:
TRICEPS

SET UP/ Sit at the very edge of a flat bench, placing your feet flat on the floor. Place your hands close to your body on the edge of the bench. Lift your weight up on your hands and slip your buttocks just in front of the bench **[A]**.

ACTION/ Lower your buttocks down close to the floor by bending your elbows **[B]**. Your elbows will want to flare out, but try to keep them close to your body. Push your body back up by straightening your arms.

ADVANCED/ Lift your feet up onto another bench and perform the same movement.

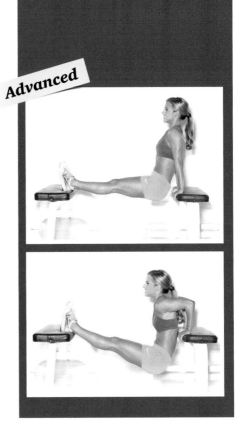

Advanced

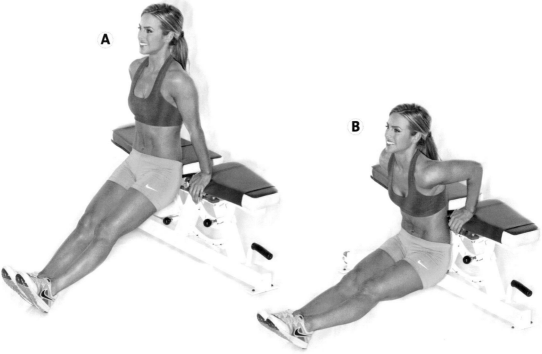

A

B

10// *Hammer Curls with a Twist*

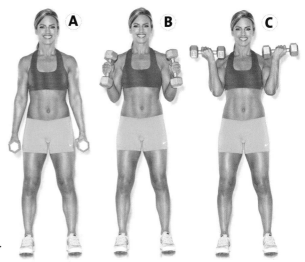

TONES THESE AREAS:
BICEPS AND FOREARMS

SET UP/ Stand, feet shoulder-width apart and knees slightly bent, holding a dumbbell in each hand at arm's length, palms facing in **[A]**.

ACTION/ Keeping your upper arms stationary, bend your elbows to bring the weights toward your shoulders, keeping your palms facing each other the entire time **[B]**. At the top, turn your hands so the dumbbells face your shoulders **[C]**. Return to the start and repeat.

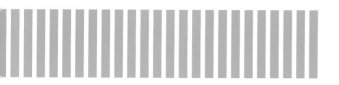

11// *Front Presses*

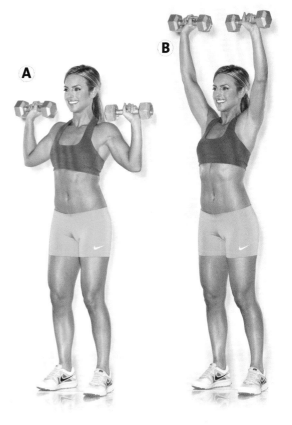

TONES THESE AREAS:
FRONT DELTOIDS (SHOULDERS)

SET UP/ Stand, feet shoulder-width apart, holding two dumbbells at shoulder height **[A]**.

ACTION/ Holding your midsection in tight, press the dumbbells toward the ceiling, bringing them together at the top **[B]**. Lower to the shoulders and repeat.

12// *Laterals*

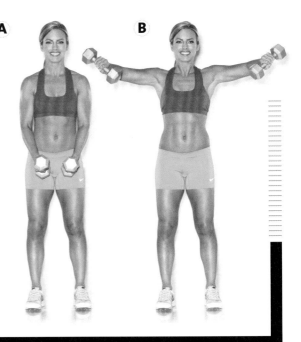

A   B

TONES THESE AREAS:
SIDE DELTOIDS (SHOULDERS)

SET UP/ Stand, feet shoulder-width apart, holding two dumbbells in front of your thighs, arms slightly bent **[A]**.

ACTION/ Keeping your elbows bent, raise your arms out to the sides **[B]**. Lead the movement with your elbows, up to shoulder height and back down. Repeat.

13// *Rear Laterals*

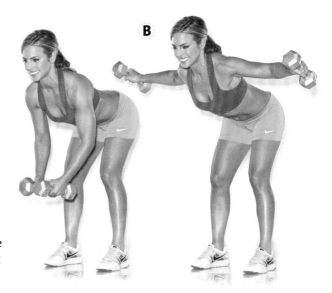

A   B

TONES THESE AREAS:
REAR DELTOIDS (SHOULDERS)

SET UP/ Stand, feet shoulder-width apart, holding two dumbbells. Bend over at the hip, keeping your back straight or arched, holding the dumbbells toward the floor with elbows slightly bent **[A]**.

ACTION/ Keeping your core tight, your back straight and your arms bent at the same angle throughout, pull the weights up to the sides, level with your back **[B]**. They should stay in line with your shoulders throughout the movement up and back down.

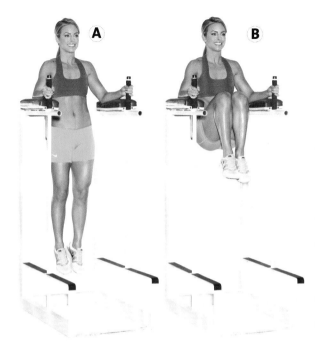

14// *Captain's Chair*

TONES THESE AREAS:
ABDOMINALS

SET UP/ Stand at the captain's chair apparatus, forearms resting on the arms, holding the handles. Lift yourself up and press your back against the backrest, letting your legs hang **[A]**.

ACTION/ Holding yourself up with your back pressed against the backrest, lift your knees toward your chest **[B]** and then lower them back down. Repeat.

ADVANCED/ Instead of lifting your knees, keep your legs straight and lift your legs toward your chest.

15// *Captain's Chair Obliques*

TONES THESE AREAS:
ABDOMINALS

SET UP/ Stand at the captain's chair apparatus, forearms resting on the arms, holding the handles. Lift yourself up and press your back against the backrest, letting your legs hang **[A]**.

ACTION/ Holding yourself up with your back pressed against the backrest, bring your knees up and to the right side **[B]**. Bring your legs down and repeat the motion on your left side **[C]**. Continue.

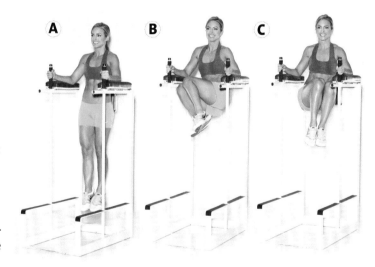

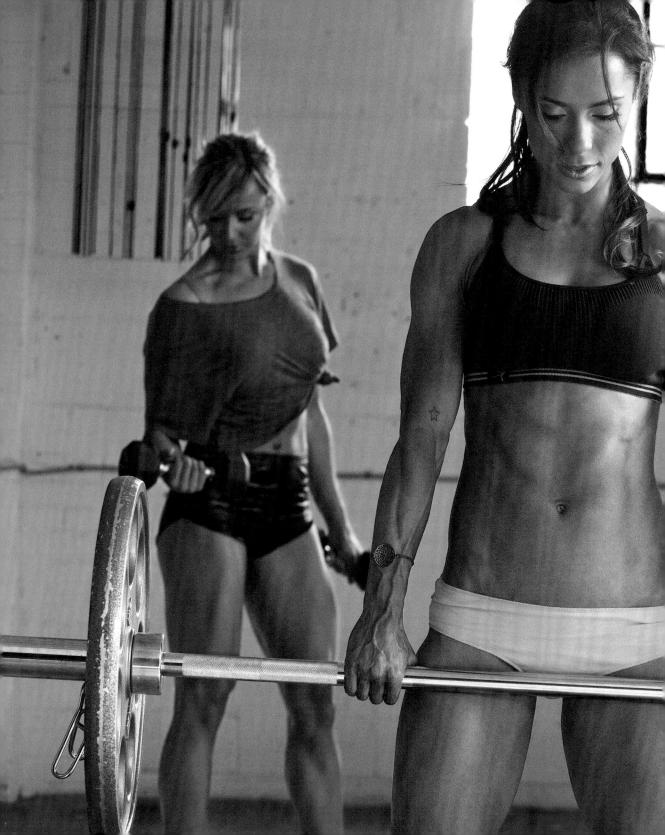

Secrets of the Sisters in Iron

THESE SIMPLE WORKOUT TIPS FROM *OXYGEN*'S FITNESS MODELS WILL HELP YOU GET (AND STAY) SLEEK AND STRONG!

"Targeting the abductors and adductors can be tough, so at the end of my treadmill workouts, I do two to three sets of one-minute interval 'side-step shuffles' right on the track, using an incline of 1.5 to 2 and a speed of around 3.5 mph. Burn, baby, burn!"
— NATALIE WAPLES

"I usually center my diet around the type of training I'm doing that day. On lifting days I pack in the protein and keep carbs low, but on a long-distance canyon run, I pack in the healthy carbs to keep my energy levels up."
— AMBER ELIZABETH

"I've consciously made my health a priority, so I schedule my workouts ahead of time and don't allow excuses. I also write down exactly what workout I will do so when I get there I can get right down to business. On days that I'm short on time, I plan a circuit or superset workout and keep the pace fast."
— PATTY ZARIELLO

"Training glutes is the one sure thing you can do to keep your metabolism (and your back end) from sliding completely into the toilet with advancing age."
— TOSCA RENO

"After a decade of living the Oxygen lifestyle, I've learned the trick is to keep myself from getting bored with my workouts and falling into a recipe rut. I created a binder full of new training ideas and easy recipes that keep my eating and training fresh and exciting."
— KIM DOLAN LETO

"Change one of the following every six to eight weeks: Frequency of workouts (e.g., four times per week instead of three), intensity of workout (level eight on the elliptical instead of level six), length of time of workout (60 minutes instead of 45 minutes) and type of workout (pull-ups instead of lat pull-downs, etc.). This is known as the F.I.T.T. principle – a must, since your body will plateau and adapt over the course of a couple of months. Varying your workouts is key to shocking your system and reaching your fitness goals quicker!"
— KAREN-LISA BORDERS

Fitness Models
RACHEL DAVIS (LEFT)**, ANDREIA BRAZIER** (CENTER) **AND ERICA WILLICK**

Navigating the Gym

Some days it can be hard enough getting to the gym, let alone trying to figure out all of the unspoken rules once you get there. Don't stress! With this guide you'll be able to keep your sweating to the workout and not over whether or not you've committed a major faux pas! *(PS. If you think this guide applies only to newbies, think again! Sometimes even hardcore gym-goers need a little freshening up)*.

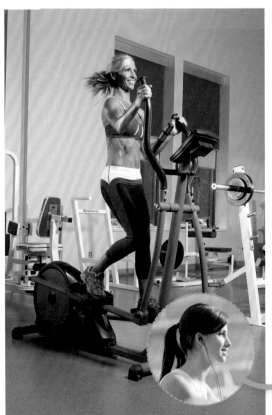

Ditch the anxiety.
Remember that you belong here just as much as those beefcakes do. If you're worried about how to use the equipment, get a friend or personal trainer to show you the ropes. Of course, you can also refer to this book and the pages of *Oxygen* for training routines and examples of correct form.

Practice safe smells.
Apply antiperspirant liberally, but ditch the perfume and cologne.

Leave your cell phone in lockup.
Many gyms are cell-phone-free zones. This not only saves members from having to listen to endless gabbing, it is also an issue of security and privacy.

Be kind to your eardrums.
Don't worry, Toto's "Africa" will still get you pumped at a volume that won't annoy the person working out beside you.

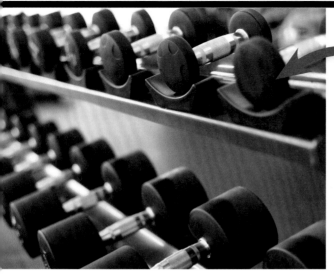

Put your weights back.

Because A) weights that have been left on the floor are a tripping hazard, and B) nothing disrupts your flow like having to hunt for a missing dumbbell that someone was too lazy to put back … or having to hoist 45-pound plates off a machine you want to use.

Watch where you walk.

If you're walking in front of a mirror, make sure you aren't blocking the view of someone who is using it to check his or her form.

Be on time.

If you're going to be late for a group class, then you should probably just catch the next session. Tardiness is disruptive and you'll have probably missed the warmup anyway.

Don't sneak out.

Try to avoid leaving class early. If you have to do it, though, mention it to your instructor beforehand (otherwise he or she may wonder if you are injured or if the class has been sub-par). Try not to disrupt your fellow students when you leave, but be sure to return your mats/equipment and wipe down your bike.

Shh!

Yes, another rule that will give you flashbacks to public school: Don't talk while class is in session – you won't get sent to the principal's office, but you will definitely get some dirty looks.

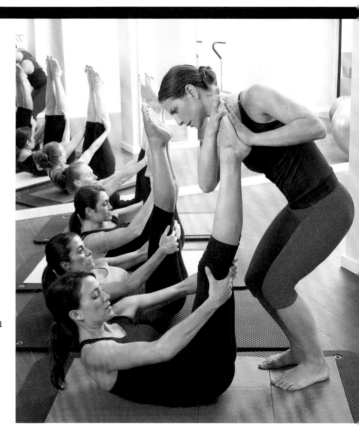

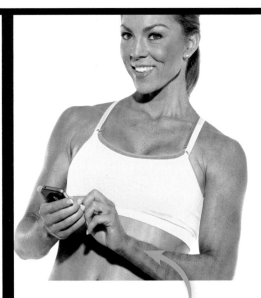

Be considerate.

Don't monopolize the equipment by lounging on machines between your sets. Whenever possible, let other members work in (alternate sets with you). Also, if your cardio equipment has a time limit, be sure to observe it – especially during peak hours.

Don't be *that* person.

Sure you've learned a lot and you want to share, but unless you see someone at risk of seriously injuring herself, it is best to avoid offering unsolicited advice to your fellow gym-goers.

Towel time!

Sweating is sexy, and so is the act of wiping sweat off of equipment with either a towel from home or one that's provided by your gym. You can also place a towel on the bench before you sit on it, to prevent leaving sweat pools. Most gyms these days have a cleaning spray plus paper towels, so there's no excuse!

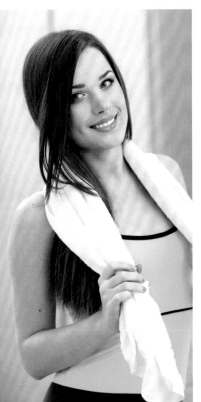

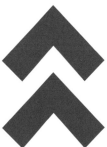

No call is that important.

Keep that cell phone in your gym bag – especially in the change room (Unless, of course, you want people to think you're covertly filming their disrobing routine).

Modesty is the best policy.

We know you've worked hard on your body, but for the comfort of others, it's best to keep it covered up with a towel. Carrying on a conversation with a nude stranger is not most people's favorite pastime.

Don't monopolize the shower.

Save water and the sanity of those around you by doing a quick wash 'n' go. Also, don't let the shower run endlessly to "warm up" while you are off doing other things. This will only succeed in getting your fellow gym-goers (not to mention the gym owner) steamed.

Invest in shower shoes.

It doesn't matter whether you choose flip-flops from the dollar store or fancy aqua socks, the gym is the one place where shoes in the shower are a definite must.

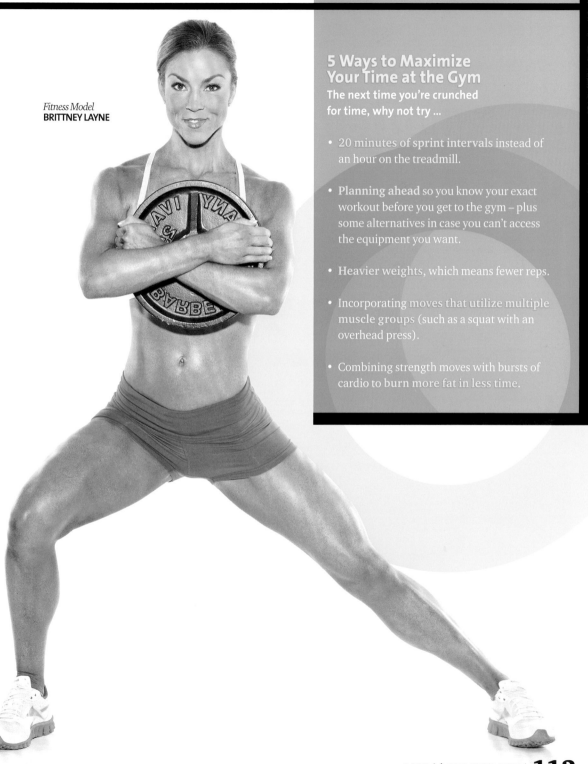

Fitness Model
BRITTNEY LAYNE

5 Ways to Maximize Your Time at the Gym

The next time you're crunched for time, why not try …

- 20 minutes of sprint intervals instead of an hour on the treadmill.

- **Planning ahead** so you know your exact workout before you get to the gym – plus some alternatives in case you can't access the equipment you want.

- Heavier weights, which means fewer reps.

- Incorporating moves that utilize multiple muscle groups (such as a squat with an overhead press).

- Combining strength moves with bursts of cardio to burn more fat in less time.

The Oxygen Diet Solution Success Story

UNWILLING TO SETTLE FOR "AVERAGE," MITCHIE DE LEON PICKED UP WEIGHT TRAINING AND DROPPED 78 POUNDS.

"I wanted to be the best me possible!"

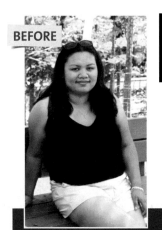

BEFORE

At 208 pounds, the last place Mitchie De Leon wanted to be was in front of a camera. But when she dropped the first 70 pounds, she was inspired to do something she'd never dreamed of: Mitchie scheduled a beach photo shoot and strutted in front of the lens in celebration.

BEFORE: 208 lb
NOW: 130 lb
AGE: 33
HEIGHT: 5'6"
LOCATION: Long Beach, CA
OCCUPATION: Event planner
FAVORITE EXERCISE: Boxing and riding her bike along the beach!

Hello, weights

On her first days in the gym's free-weights area, Mitchie didn't feel comfortable and roped a guy pal into accompanying her. "When I did chest presses on a flat bench using dumb-bells, I started out with 15 pounds and thought that was heavy," Mitchie recalls. "Now, I use 40s and get looks." With a spotter, she pushes out three reps with 55s! "I changed my whole mentality about working out," says Mitchie. "I'm no longer scared."

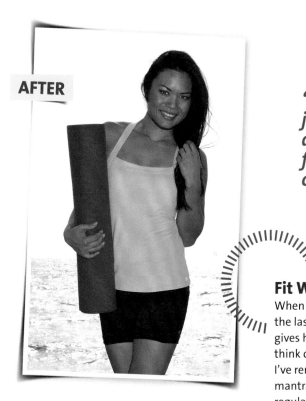

AFTER

"Having a fit body is a journey and lifestyle. It's not a quick task to accomplish for an event. It's about the choices I make daily."

Fit Words

When she's struggling to get through the last set at the gym, Mitchie gives herself personal pep talks. "I think of the motivational quotes I've remembered, almost like little mantras," she says. Three of her regulars include:

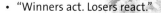

- "Winners act. Losers react."
- "Strive for progress, not perfection."
- "The only people who fail are those who don't try."

Lift-off

As an event planner, Mitchie didn't see a way around the long (and calorie-packed) client dinners until she cleaned up her diet. Watching her portions, Mitchie shed the first 50 pounds. She then got creative with exercise, moving away from the treadmill to try spinning, Body Pump and group exercise classes in addition to lifting weights. She still gets active with cardio daily. This self-proclaimed cardio queen likes to sweat! Inspired by the physiques of fitness models in *Oxygen*, she entered a Bikini-division physique show.

Body Aware

One of the biggest benefits of her fat-loss transformation? Mitchie says she's become more aware of her health, fitness and, most importantly, her body. "Whenever I go to the gym or try a new workout, I learn something new about my body," she says. "I have nice biceps, for example."

Mitchie's Meals

Cleaning up some of her favorite recipes was key to Mitchie's success. Some of her favorite dinners include:

Meal 1: Ground turkey with stir-fried vegetables and Mrs. Dash in a brown rice tortilla, over brown rice or on a salad

Meal 2: Clean chicken curry with quinoa

Meal 3: Brown rice pasta or shirataki (tofu) noodles with ground turkey, peppers, tomatoes and spinach in marinara sauce

PART II

WHOLE BODY HEALTH

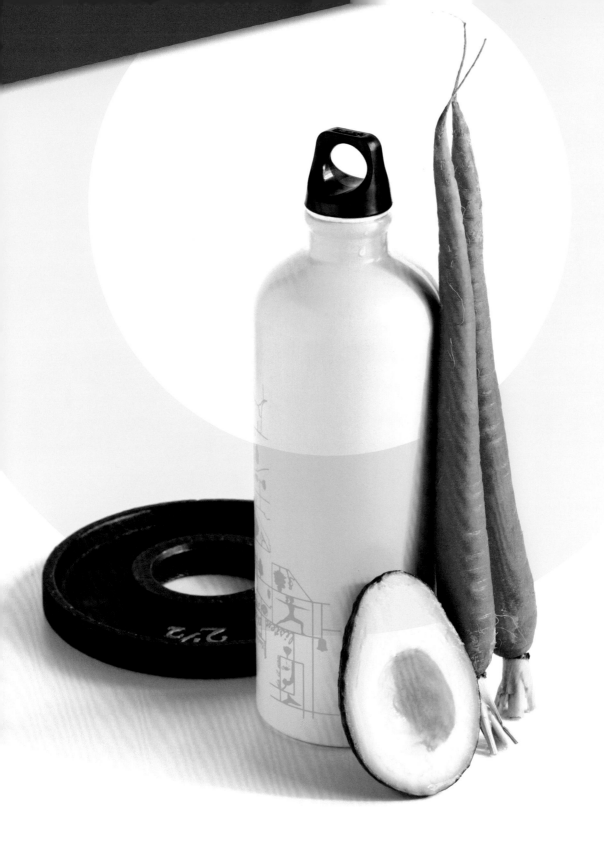

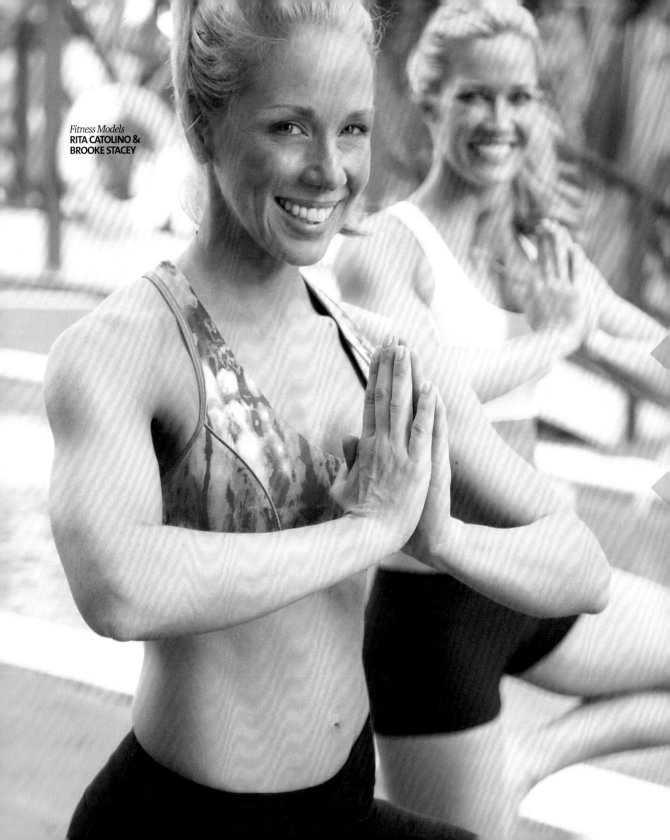

Healthy Body, Healthy Mind

Beat stress, boost confidence and enjoy life to the fullest

You make an effort to choose healthy foods, you work out five days a week and you try to squeeze in some family time whenever you can, but you still feel like you're stuck in a rut. Chances are you're also tired, overwhelmed, stretched too many ways and feeling lethargic. If this sounds familiar, your problem may lie in the fact that you're not treating your mind with the same health-consciousness you devote to your body – and that just won't do!

Stress and worrying take a toll on your wellbeing, from your mindset to your physical self to how you react with others, but it's often hard to stop all the worrying. Remember that you can change the outcome of a situation by actively choosing how you'll approach it, and then how you'll respond to it after. When you worry about an event, your body reacts as if the event has already happened. In effect, the more often you worry about a specific outcome, the more times you have to go through the exact event you're worrying about!

Many women out there don't realize the impact an overworked and underappreciated mind can have on their overall health. When your head is full of negative thoughts, even the smallest glitch can throw off your whole day. Yes, your stressed brain will still let you perform your usual 20 minutes of HIIT, but if you are obsessing over a bygone incident with a rude cashier or coworker, you will A) not be getting the most out of your workout and B) not be enjoying your life.

So what are you waiting for? It's time to take that extra step and look after your mind as well as your body. Get out of the worry habit for the good of your physical health and your peace of mind. You'll be amazed at how a healthy outlook can supercharge your weight-loss journey – and your life!

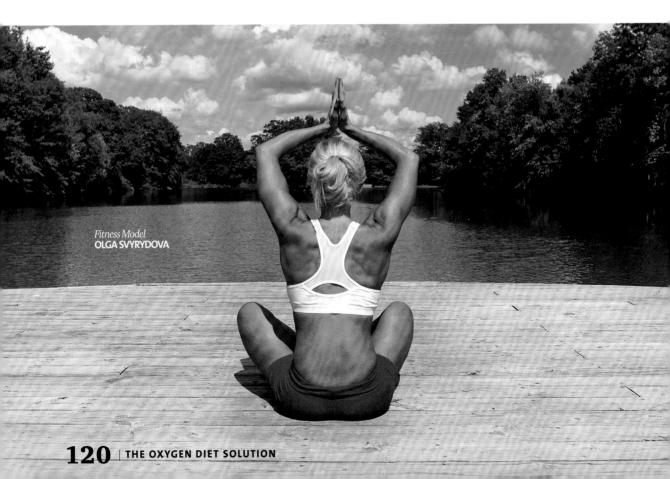

Fitness Model
OLGA SVYRYDOVA

5 STRESS-BUSTING FOODS

WALNUTS – Walnuts and walnut oil have been found to lower blood-pressure responses to stress. While foods can't change your emotional response to stress, they can change your physiological response, says Sheila G. West, PhD, associate professor of behavioral health and nutritional sciences at Pennsylvania State University. To get the benefits, consume 1½ ounces of walnuts or 1 tbsp of walnut oil daily.

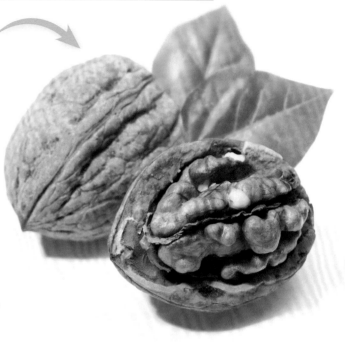

SALMON – The omega-3 fatty acids found in fatty fish such as salmon have been shown to reduce heart rate during times of stress, which is good news for anyone feeling overwhelmed. Healthy adults can enjoy two to five meals of fatty fish a week, or one gram of fish oil daily. Arctic char, black cod, fresh albacore tuna, halibut, mackerel, rainbow trout, herring, sardines, anchovies, oysters and mussels are some more good options.

BANANAS – Potassium-rich foods such as bananas and potatoes can help reduce blood pressure caused by stress, since potassium is known for controlling blood pressure and heart function. To keep your blood pressure within a healthy range and protect your heart, include one potassium source daily to reap the benefits.

ORANGES – Oranges are known for their vitamin C content, but did you know about vitamin C's ability to reduce the secretion of the stress hormone cortisol? Include an orange, some strawberries, cantaloupe or red pepper in your daily diet to fight the effects of cortisol. This stress hormone also makes the body store fat, especially in the abdominal area.

DARK LEAFY GREENS – B vitamins found in dark leafy greens are great stress busters, so load up on spinach, kale and collards to leave stress in the dust. Bonus: You'll also find a range of stress-reducing B vitamins in whole grains, legumes, squash, pecans and almonds.

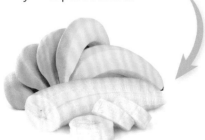

Beat Stress

Stress is caused by a number of factors – too many responsibilities, commuting woes, problems at work and family troubles, to name a few – and it manifests itself in an even greater number of unhealthy ways. You can experience symptoms ranging from fatigue, depression and memory problems to immune deficiency and mysterious aches and pains.

Although you will never be able to fully eliminate stress from your life, you can take comfort in the fact that not all stress is bad. When you feel threatened, your body sparks the fight or flight response, which is key to survival. Good stress helps you get things done. But when stress becomes chronic, that's when you need to take action. The good news? The power to beat stress is in your hands! You can learn to control your response to stressful situations, and it is your reaction to the stressors in your life that will dictate how it affects you.

Get ready to let go, loosen up and start feeling amazing with these seven simple tips.

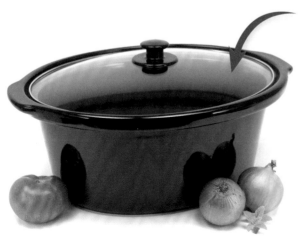

1 / Shake it out

No, we're not talking about the Hokey Pokey! Rather, a simple exercise that can help alleviate the stress of a long day. After work or a long meeting, shake out your right leg, then your left leg, right arm and left arm. Then twist your torso, roll your head and give your full body one good shake.

2 / Feel the beat

Place your fingers on your wrist or neck, feel for your pulse, and start counting. As you count, you'll feel your heart rate slow. This is because the counting not only distracts you from thinking about anything else, it also puts you in tune with your own body's rhythm, which can be soothing, says Ashley Davis Bush, a New Hampshire-based psychotherapist.

3 / Cook up some comfort

Whatever the time of year, comfort food is always a welcome reprieve from "health food," but why not have the best of both worlds? Kick up the comfort with a clean slow-cooker meal that takes absolutely no effort to put together and yet delivers on taste. (Check out *Clean Eating* magazine for tons of inspiration and recipes.) Instead of stressing about getting dinner on the table, you'll just be wondering about which delicious slow-cooker meal you should try next!

4 / Breathing 6-3-6-3

This isn't breathing 101, but it's not too far off! If you feel a meltdown coming on, try this technique: Place your tongue on the roof of your mouth, behind the hard ridge that sits behind your top row of teeth. Inhale deeply for six counts and hold for three counts, then exhale for six counts and hold for three more counts. Repeat these steps until you feel the calm roll in.

5 / Get active

Though this may seem counterintuitive, being active is a great way to relieve stress. The gym is always a sensible place to start pounding out your frustration on the treadmill, but don't discount the benefits of getting outside! Nature is one of the most relaxing, anti-stress environments out there (no pun intended). Whether you're the type to hike, canoe, kayak or cycle, interacting with nature while you work your body will also allow you to calm your mind and release any built-up stress. You may find you have to talk yourself into getting started, but make yourself a deal that you'll go for only five minutes, for example. Once you do get on your way, you'll find you have more energy than you thought you had, and you'll keep going – and feel great afterward!

To avoid letting stress get the better of you, step back from a situation and ask yourself the following questions:

- Will this situation I'm about to walk into cause me stress?

- How can I change my reaction in order to not feel stressed?

- Which steps can I take to keep calm and grounded before I let stress take over?

- How can I control my reaction so that I don't harm others around me?

Once you've learned to control your response to a stressful situation, you'll realize you can and will avoid stress in the future, and say goodbye to those negative side effects, too.

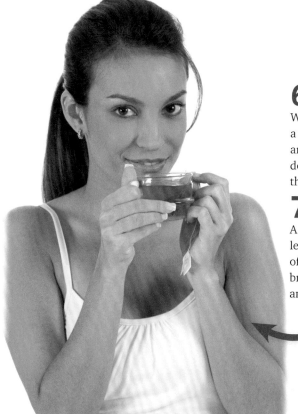

6 / DIY massage

What could be better than a massage? How about a free one! Take off your shoes, sit on the floor, and thread your fingers between your toes. As you do this, rub your feet, which will reduce tension throughout your whole body.

7 / Tea time

A cup of tea can calm not only your stress level – it can also calm your stomach. Stress often manifests itself as stomach trouble, so brew up some peppermint tea to bust stress and soothe your tummy all at once.

Live Longer and Better

Does living longer seem like something out of a science fiction story? With the right tools, the right mindset and a healthy lifestyle, it can become your reality! You can make your life both longer and of a much higher quality by staying healthy, active and fit. Staying healthy and fit will also help keep your mind sharp into your later years. Better to make the most of life now so you can appreciate it all the more – and for much longer – later!

Physical health is a must when it comes to a longer and better-quality life, but your emotional and mental health are just as important. Your mind-body connection runs much deeper than you may think; the more time and attention you devote to your mental health, the better you'll be able to achieve the goals you set for your physical health. Have you ever noticed your workouts aren't quite up to your usual standard when you're feeling tired, upset or stressed? Your mental state is affected by everything from a lack of sleep to a negative emotion or excessive responsibility – any of these distractions take away from your physical performance. Emotions such as guilt, anger or sadness can also affect your dedication to a clean diet. (Stress eating, anyone?)

It's time to step back and take a look at the aspects of your health you don't always think of so you can follow through with the goals you've set for yourself. This section is all about YOU – your health, your wellbeing, your longevity – how to make yourself feel better inside and out. So take the time to get familiar with your challenges and the strategies listed here to help you live a longer and better life.

Quick Steps to Boost Your Health

Though your genes determine many things – your hair and eye color, for instance – they do not determine how long you'll live. Sure you may be predisposed to certain diseases, but your life expectancy depends more on the day-to-day choices you make, which is where the *Oxygen* lifestyle comes in. With some simple strategies, you can boost your health now to increase your life expectancy, your quality of life and the enjoyment and fulfillment you'll get out of treating yourself right. First step? Turn off the TV.

We'll say it straight out: your TV is killing you. Don't believe us? One study found that each hour you spend sitting in front of the TV raises your risk of dying from all causes! Next time you're tempted by *Mad Men* or a *Dawson's Creek* marathon, drop the remote, lace up your shoes and go for a walk instead. You'll extend your life by leaps and bounds by not only turning off the TV, but by choosing an activity that has a proven benefit to your health.

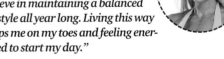

FIT TIP

"Staying on track with the Oxygen *lifestyle comes as second nature. I believe in maintaining a balanced lifestyle all year long. Living this way keeps me on my toes and feeling energized to start my day."*

– Aleisha Hart, fitness model

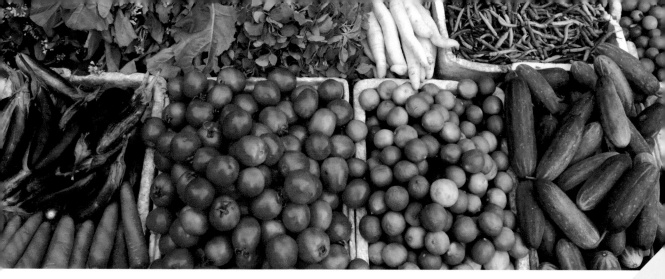

You've probably heard variety is the spice of life, but did you know it's also the breath of life? Diversifying your diet means you get a large range of disease-fighting compounds, since each type of fruit and vegetable contains different micronutrients, phytonutrients and antioxidants. For example, if you include mustard greens in your salad and have strawberries for dessert, you get compounds that lower cholesterol and antioxidants that help reduce inflammation, all in one meal.

But don't just diversify your diet – make it exotic! Try following a Mediterranean-style diet full of fruits, vegetables, beans, nuts and fish to reduce your risk of death and disease. These foods are loaded with monounsaturated and polyunsaturated fatty acids, which lower the risk of coronary heart disease.

Another simple way to improve your health through your diet is to increase your fiber intake. In one study published in the journal *Archives of Internal Medicine*, women who consumed the greatest amount of dietary fiber were up to 59 percent less likely to die during a nine-year period than those who ate the least fiber. Aim for 25 to 35 grams daily from whole foods, but if you're having trouble sneaking enough fiber into your meals, consider adding a supplement.

You should also go nuts – no, really! An ounce of nuts per day can boost your health. Each kind of nut delivers different nutrient benefits, so be sure to mix it up. Walnuts contain large amounts of antioxidants, for example, while pecans are said to protect against LDL (or "bad") cholesterol.

Get more of your protein from nuts, too – and other vegetarian, fish and white-meat sources. Reducing red meat in your diet will help protect your heart, according to a study published in *Archives of Internal Medicine*, which found that women who ate the most red meat were 50 percent more likely to die from heart disease over a 10-year period than those who ate the least. Try limiting your red meat intake to less than 18 ounces (or about four servings) per week, and choose the leanest possible cuts.

Another way to avoid an early death is to build strong bones. Strengthening your bones helps prevent osteoporosis, as well as fractures in later life that can lead to an early death. Your best defense against these bone-shattering scares is to get at least 600 IU of vitamin D, 1,000 mg of calcium and 320 mg of magnesium daily. Since dosage varies with age, as a general rule aim for a ratio of 2:1 calcium to magnesium to get maximum nutrient absorption.

Now that you feel strong, it's easier to be positive. Postmenopausal women who are optimistic are 14 percent less likely to die from any cause, and 30 percent less likely to die from coronary heart disease, than their pessimistic counterparts. Optimism will lead to happiness, being happy will make you laugh and laughing can decrease levels of the stress hormones cortisol and adrenaline, which cause inflammation in the body and increase your risk of disease. Avoid disease by laughing off something you would normally have taken to heart, or laugh at yourself instead of stressing the next time you make a mistake. Now that's what you call the power of positivity!

Get Fit From the Inside

Don't forget about the importance of getting fit from the inside out when it comes to living longer! Your organs work extremely hard each day to keep you healthy, fit and strong. Pay them back by taking the best care of them possible.

Your brain and heart are two of the key players in your body's internal function, so they need extra TLC to stay in top shape. Boost your brain power and heart health by getting active. Each time you exercise, you increase the flow of oxygen to your brain, which can lead to improved memory, focus and clarity. Meanwhile, your heart keeps all your other organs functioning properly, since it pumps oxygenated blood throughout your body. It needs 30 minutes of cardiovascular exercise five or six days a week at 65 to 70 percent or more of your maximum heart rate. The more fit you are, the more blood your heart can pump per beat, meaning it doesn't have to work as hard to distribute the blood throughout your body.

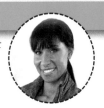

Cardiovascular exercise will also strengthen your lungs, which perform the vital function of bringing in oxygen for your heart to distribute! You can also strengthen your lung function by training your core with yoga or Pilates, since these moves engage the muscles in your diaphragm. You will not be surprised that we suggest avoiding both direct and secondhand smoke, which can irritate the airways, cause inflammation and damage cells in the lungs, but you may be surprised to hear that smoking is responsible for about one in five deaths in the US, and about 80 percent of all lung cancer deaths in women. Not only does smoking lead to early death, it also causes premature aging. In fact, among other negative effects, smoking inhibits your oxygen supply, which affects every cell in your body – even your skin.

The other supportive players in your overall health are your kidneys and liver. Hydration is key in their care and maintenance; your kidneys need lots of water to let them balance your blood minerals and electrolytes, preventing cramps and muscle soreness, and your liver needs plenty of water since it is a crucial part of your body's cleansing system, allowing for detoxification, protein synthesis and production of digestive chemicals. To keep your liver clean, aim for two to three liters of water daily and avoid alcohol, which is toxic to the liver and can lead to inflammation and scarring. Keeping your triglyceride levels low with a clean diet low in refined carbohydrates is also a good way to avoid a fatty liver, and in turn avoid damaging its cells.

Make Time for Yourself

This wouldn't be a complete section on living better if we didn't recommend a little bit of "you" time. It's important to take time not only to relax, but also to find balance, get in touch with your inner self and enjoy the company of the people you love most – including your friends! With these strategies, you'll focus on your mental and emotional health to improve your quality of life – and the enjoyment you get from it. We'll drink (a clean cocktail) to that!

Yoga

You've heard about the benefits of yoga, but have you ever really heeded them? Yoga is a great way to take care of both your physical and mental health. Talk about a two-fer! There's nothing more peaceful than spending an hour getting in touch with your inner self by channeling your physical strength into challenging poses. You'll learn about your physical boundaries, yes, but you'll also learn what it takes to mentally push yourself to complete the sequence. **Turn to p. 84 for a relaxing beginning to yoga.**

Spa day with the girls

Sometimes what you need to relax and get back in touch with your inner self is a manicure, pedicure and the company of your girlfriends. Plan an at-home spa day with three of your closest friends so you can each have a turn sitting back and getting pampered.

Try giving each other manicures, pedicures, massages and facials. Stick with naturally derived products for a relaxing experience that won't cause problems to your health, your skin or the environment. Even better, do your manicure and pedicure with just some massaging or exfoliating cream and cuticle oil – go without nail polish for a more natural look and feel.

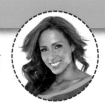
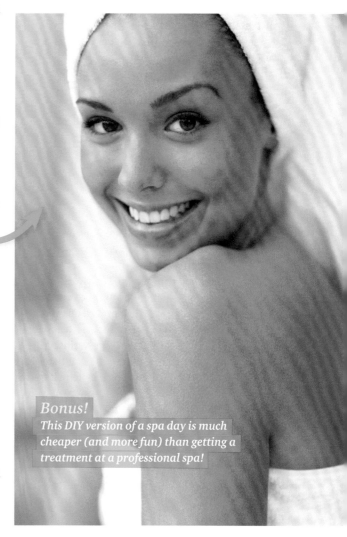

Bonus!
This DIY version of a spa day is much cheaper (and more fun) than getting a treatment at a professional spa!

VIRGIN STRAWBERRY MARGARITA

Ready in 10 minutes
Makes 4 servings

2 cups fresh or frozen strawberries
1 lime, juiced
2 tbsp raw honey
12 oz water
12 ice cubes
12 mint leaves, to garnish

1. Place strawberries, lime, honey and half of the water in a blender. Blend thoroughly.

2. Add ice and remaining water gradually to reach desired consistency. Add more ice if desired.

Nutrients per serving (10 oz):
Calories: 60, Total Fats: 0 g, Saturated Fat: 0 g, Trans Fat: 0 g, Cholesterol: 0 mg, Sodium: 8 mg, Total Carbohydrates: 16 g, Dietary Fiber: 2 g, Sugars: 14 g, Protein: 0 g, Iron: 1 mg

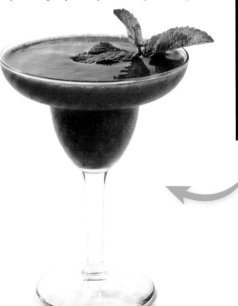

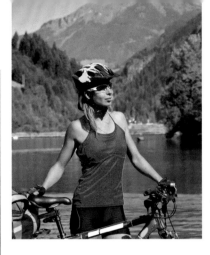

Try a new activity

A great way to grow and change – and find something new to enjoy! – is to step outside your usual boundaries. Trying a new activity is a great way to learn about yourself, especially how you react in new situations. Whether you attempt a Zumba class or take up extreme mountain biking, you'll learn more about yourself than you would simply sitting back and doing your usual thing. Take it slow to test your boundaries and find out if your new activity is something you'll want to stick with, or if you'll have better luck with something else.

Girls' night in ... or out

Kicking back with your girlfriends may be just the thing you need to unwind after a long day of work. Try watching a movie, dishing the latest gossip and enjoying some clean eats while you're at it! Choose a comedy if you're looking to burn off some steam – laughter is the best medicine, after all.

To make it a true girls' night, try whipping up some clean virgin strawberry margaritas (see sidebar) to accompany all the girl talk. This divine drink will make you feel like you're at an upscale lounge instead of just lounging in your sweats!

Want a little more excitement? Try a girls' night out! Whether you go dancing, bowling or simply take a dinner tour from one friend's house to the next, keep it clean and active so you don't have to feel guilty about a bit of overindulgence.

Boost your Energy

You get up, get dressed, make sure the kids are up, put the coffee on, eat breakfast and pack the lunches – all by 7 am! No wonder most women are so drained. You need to kick your energy into high gear so you can successfully tackle your day – and keep your emotional health running strong. More energy means you'll have a more positive outlook, you'll feel happier all day and you're more likely to end it on a high note.

Start your day off right by choosing to work out as your day begins, rather than waiting until later in the day when excuses and delays can get in the way of your resolve. Morning exercise is a great energy booster; accomplishing something first thing starts your day off on a positive note, and your thinking becomes clearer for the day ahead. As a bonus, research from Appalachian State University suggests exercising within an hour of waking results in better-quality sleep than exercising in the afternoon or evening. That means those morning sweat sessions are actually helping you get up early – the better the sleep you get, the better the quality of exercise the next morning. What a great cycle!

The quality of your sleep is essential, but don't forget about the quantity! Getting plenty of sleep is crucial to keeping up your energy during the day. Though it's tempting to have a late dinner if you get home from work late or have an after-dinner coffee when you have dinner guests, the effects of a late dinner or snack can have a huge impact on the length and quality of your sleep. The caffeine in coffee is an obvious stimulant, but don't forget about the effort it takes your body to digest a meal – if you're trying to hit the hay right when your body is working hard to assimilate all the nutrients you've given it, chances are you'll have trouble drifting off and staying asleep. Instead, try an earlier dinner (at least four hours before your bedtime), and avoid coffee any later than 3 pm to ensure it doesn't affect your sleep later on.

FIT TIP

"One of the biggest motivators for me is knowing what life without achievement and goals feels like. Now I know the things that bring you the most satisfaction are the things that are the hardest to do. It usually involves facing a fear or having to sacrifice some things, but it always ends up bringing the greatest rewards in the end."

– Lori Harder, fitness model

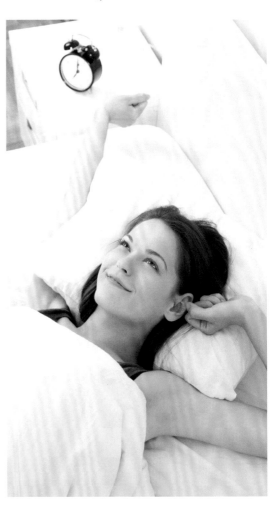

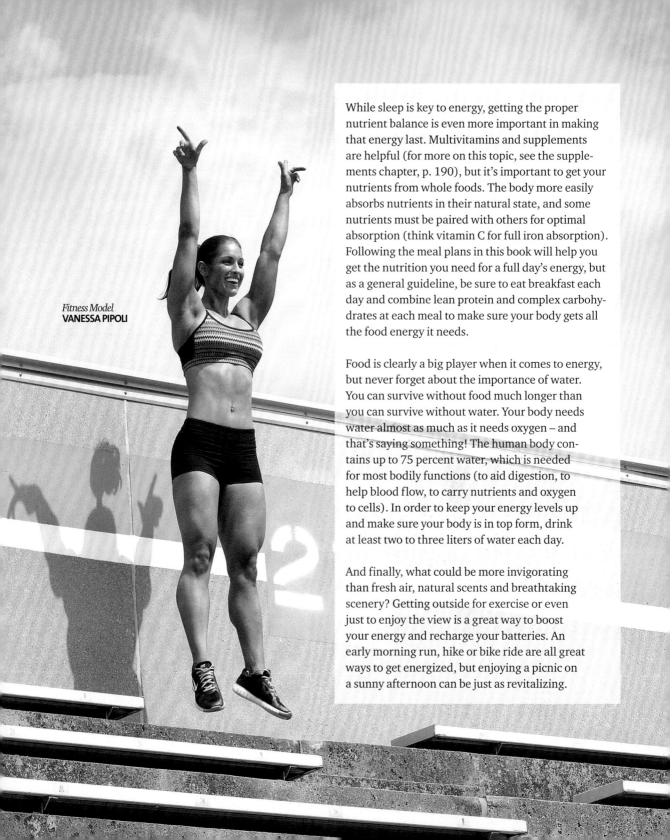

Fitness Model
VANESSA PIPOLI

While sleep is key to energy, getting the proper nutrient balance is even more important in making that energy last. Multivitamins and supplements are helpful (for more on this topic, see the supplements chapter, p. 190), but it's important to get your nutrients from whole foods. The body more easily absorbs nutrients in their natural state, and some nutrients must be paired with others for optimal absorption (think vitamin C for full iron absorption). Following the meal plans in this book will help you get the nutrition you need for a full day's energy, but as a general guideline, be sure to eat breakfast each day and combine lean protein and complex carbohydrates at each meal to make sure your body gets all the food energy it needs.

Food is clearly a big player when it comes to energy, but never forget about the importance of water. You can survive without food much longer than you can survive without water. Your body needs water almost as much as it needs oxygen – and that's saying something! The human body contains up to 75 percent water, which is needed for most bodily functions (to aid digestion, to help blood flow, to carry nutrients and oxygen to cells). In order to keep your energy levels up and make sure your body is in top form, drink at least two to three liters of water each day.

And finally, what could be more invigorating than fresh air, natural scents and breathtaking scenery? Getting outside for exercise or even just to enjoy the view is a great way to boost your energy and recharge your batteries. An early morning run, hike or bike ride are all great ways to get energized, but enjoying a picnic on a sunny afternoon can be just as revitalizing.

Energy By The Numbers

25

The percentage that your fatigue will be reduced by if you sniff some peppermint. (Try brewing up some minty tea.)

2/3

THE ESTIMATED PORTION OF THE AMERICAN POPULATION THAT DOESN'T DRINK ENOUGH WATER, WHICH CAN LEAD TO DEHYDRATION — **A HUGE DRAIN ON ENERGY**

1.4

micrograms of energy-boosting vitamin B12 found in a 3-oz serving of lean beef — that's 23 percent of your recommended daily value.

65

percentage by which sleep quality improved in people who exercised at least 150 minutes a week, in a study from Oregon State University

27

THE GRAMS OF SUGAR IN AN 8.5-OZ CAN OF RED BULL ENERGY DRINK

Attitude is Everything

In order to achieve your healthy body and healthy mind, you have to be open to the possibility of change. Sometimes it can be scary thinking about how different things will be once you're on your journey to fit and healthy, but you must be ready for success. Here are some ways you can make over your mindset to ensure you're ready to embrace all of the positive changes that will be coming your way. Soon, you'll be so pumped to see just what you're capable of that you'll leave all worry and uncertainty in the dust!

Make Over your Gym Mindset

Success starts with being positive, so to get in the habit of positive thoughts, try celebrating and appreciating your little successes in the gym. Keep a fitness journal and write down one or two positive thoughts about the day's workout: "My legs felt strong," or "I upped the amount of weight I can press."

A quick and simple way to get back to a positive mindset is to write down your goals and post them up in places you'll easily see them. When you're feeling down, take a look at the goals you've written down and visualize how awesome you'll feel once you reach them. No one can take that feeling away from you, so be proud of yourself even before you've hit your end goal! Learn more about goal setting in the motivation chapter, p. 146.

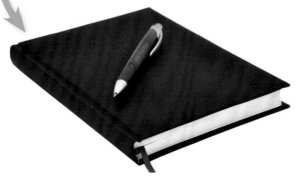

Be confident in the process rather than disappointed in the setbacks. When you feel intimidated by the big hulking men and trim and toned ladies at the gym, remember that these people are all at a different point in their fit journeys. They were all beginners once, so be confident that you too will reach your goals in due time. If you hit a snag along the way, know that you'll get past it, get back on track toward your goals and even be able to offer support and encouragement to other newbies.

Finding your inspiration is a key component to getting past those starting-out jitters. If you're in an environment where you can't get comfortable or you don't feel confident, you'll have a harder time believing in yourself and gathering the tools you need to see success. In order to reach your goals, find the right circumstances to motivate you. An environment where you feel confident and supported will be the most suitable for you. Surround yourself with like-minded people who not only encourage you, but also value the importance of a healthy lifestyle. Studies show we tend to follow the examples of those we surround ourselves with, so if your friends have healthy habits you are more likely to have healthy habits as well.

5 Quick Switches

Is your mind holding you back? Make these mindset switches now to break out of those negative thought patterns and move toward the success that comes with the right attitude!

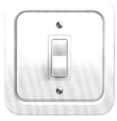

1 / The Holdup:

You're not following through with your goals. You look for and accept excuses to skip workouts or to choose unhealthy foods; there's always something getting in the way of you shopping for healthy, whole foods.

The Switch: Make appointments with yourself – book the time to make your health and fitness goals a priority. An appointment book or electronic calendar will help you organize these appointments. Book times to go to the gym and even to grocery shop for the foods in your meal plan. Write down how these healthy foods will help you reach your goals so you'll have the incentive you need to reach for them instead of junk food.

2 / The Holdup:
You keep your health and weight-loss goals to yourself. You never record your goals, perhaps because you're afraid to create accountability around them in case you fail.

The Switch: Write down your goals, but also keep focused on the steps you take each day to reach them. Every day is made up of a series of little goals: Say "no" to the donuts during your morning meeting; go for a walk at lunch hour. These accomplishments help you see the daily process behind reaching an ultimate goal, making it that much more attainable.

3 / The Holdup:
You get easily overwhelmed because you dive into weight-loss programs and diets without all the facts. You try to make too many changes at once, so you get frustrated and give up.

The Switch: Instead of that "all or nothing" attitude, try thinking incrementally. It is much easier to maintain a plan when you're celebrating and building on small successes rather than jumping in feet first and feeling smothered by too many demands and expectations you've placed on yourself.

4 / The Holdup:
Self-sabotage gets the better of you – in the form of a junk food binge, staying up late the night before a planned workout or not eating all day and then overdoing it later.

The Switch: Recognize this pattern of behavior for what it is – sabotage. Realize how it's holding you back from reaching your goals, and take the steps to protect against it, such as cleaning out your cupboards and replacing junk food with whole foods. Don't give yourself the opportunity to undermine your efforts. A fresh start is a great tool for changing your thinking.

5 / The Holdup:
You bash yourself with negative self-talk, such as "I'm fat," "I'm so ugly" or "I'll never look like that fit woman over there."

The Switch: Take care to notice the kind of language you use when talking about yourself, and make a conscious effort to reframe it in a positive way. Be your own friend. You would never speak to a friend in a negative way. Instead of saying you're fat and ugly, tell yourself you are strong, beautiful and capable of achieving anything. What you believe yourself to be, you will be, so believe yourself to be the incredible person you are.

Boost your Confidence

Confidence is king and if you want to have it, you have to believe in yourself all the way! Here are three strategies for finding and strengthening your self-confidence to ensure you meet your goals.

Strategy 1: Harness your emotions

Emotions can often be the reason you give up on something – if you feel shame or guilt about your body image, you may lose your drive to improve it. Use your emotions for good instead – have pride in your body and the motivation to work out will follow naturally, along with the confidence to see it through. Bask in the feeling of accomplishment every single time you complete a workout or eat a meal that nourishes you. It's an awesome cycle, not a vicious one!

Your Emotional Tools

Affirm your pride by getting control of the emotions that surround your body. Think of all the amazing things your body can do! Say to yourself, "I am proud of my body." Simply saying that will lay the groundwork for pride.

Banish shame by focusing on the things you are achieving rather than the things you're not achieving. This will help eliminate shame in your "shortcomings" and promote a feeling of pride in your achievements instead. No one is able to do everything she wants to immediately – we all have to work toward achieving our accomplishments, one step at a time.

Choose an empowering mantra that will boost you up instead of negative talk that will wear you down. Something as simple as "I can do this!" will switch your negative thoughts over to positive ones, and you'll feel better about yourself immediately.

Strategy 2: Look at the big picture

Though your fitness goals are important, remember they are only one part of the bigger picture. It's important to work your fitness goals into the other aspects of your life so you can achieve balance as you move toward the overarching goal of being healthy.

Your Goal-Setting Tools

Start high: Define and write down one or several "high-level" goals, such as maintaining a healthy weight for life. This high-level goal is important because it is something you will practice over a long period of time and focus all your short- and long-term efforts on.

Take the credo "Tomorrow is another day" to heart – it's easier to forgive yourself in the context of your high-level goal if you slip up, because you're going to be working toward it for the long haul. If you make a mistake one day, simply get back on plan the next to ensure you hit your short-term, medium-term and long-term targets. Success comes from what we do regularly, not from what we do once.

Change your thinking. Train yourself to think long term, because it is often hard to see progress from one day to the next. When you look back at your fitness efforts from a month ago and realize you're now lifting 10 pounds heavier, you start to see the substantial progress you've made, even if you can't see it during every workout.

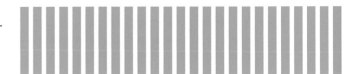

Strategy 3: Visualize your potential

Though you may think fear is an excellent motivator, positive visualization can be just as effective – or even more so. Rather than visualizing yourself as overweight, with a lethargic, sedentary lifestyle in order to scare yourself away from that outcome, try visualizing yourself with a healthy, fit lifestyle in order to move toward it. As an added bonus, positive visualization is better for your short-term happiness than fear, so you'll be thinking positive now and later!

Your Visualization Tools

Act out the future. Seeing yourself now as the person you want to be down the road will help you take the steps toward reaching that healthy, fit lifestyle.

If you don't have a plan to get back on track after a slip-up, you're more likely to fall into a negative thought pattern and have trouble getting back into your routine. Plan to start fresh if you fall off track so your positive thoughts can get you back in the groove.

Never give up! Even if you don't see chiseled abs and a toned derriere in the first week, stick with it. Visualizing your future self will offer the motivation you need to continue on your fit journey and reach all your goals – starting with short term and ending in total success!

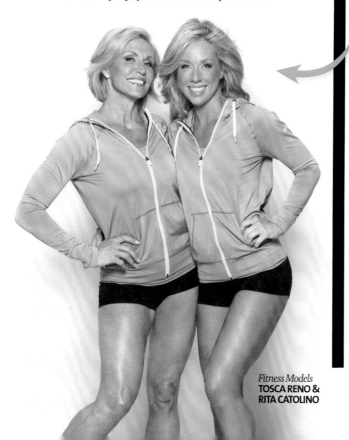

Fitness Models
**TOSCA RENO &
RITA CATOLINO**

SMILE BIG (AND MEAN IT)!

Not only does smiling make you happier – it also has proven health benefits. The only drawback: it has to be a genuine smile. If you're having trouble getting happy, start out by faking a smile. A fake smile leads to real happiness, which will lead to a real smile! Here are five ways smiling can boost your health and wellness:

1. Smiling brings about a more POSITIVE ATTITUDE.

2. Flashing a genuine smile boosts your IMMUNE SYSTEM.

3. Smiling lowers your BLOOD PRESSURE.

4. You release NATURAL PAINKILLERS in your body when you smile.

5. A simple smile can lower your STRESS LEVELS.

BONUS!

A big, deep belly laugh can help you live longer! A study from the University of Maryland School of Medicine found that watching a comedy expanded participants' blood vessel lining, improving their blood flow and potentially helping reduce the risk of heart disease.

Fit Pregnancy

Whether you're already well on your way to a fit pregnancy or you're still getting the hang of working out and eating clean, here's your go-to guide for what to eat, how to train and which products will make your pregnancy that much easier. You'll also find all the info you need for staying fit and saving time post-pregnancy, too.

Your Fit Pregnancy FAQ

Q / **Which tweaks should I make to my pre-workout routine during pregnancy?**

A: You'll need more of the following three things: food, water and warming up! Before you hit the gym, make sure your body is fueled properly.

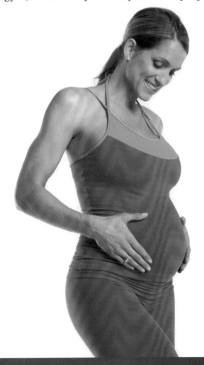

Moms-to-be need an additional 20 to 300 calories per day in their second and third trimesters. And you need to account for the calories you burn, too! Aim for lean proteins and healthy grains, fruits and veggies. Drink water before, during and after your workout to prevent dehydration. Once you begin, add a slow warm-up, like a walk, to get all those achy joints moving. Always talk to your healthcare provider about your pregnancy workouts.

Q / **Are there any danger signs I should look for if I'm working out while pregnant?**

A: You should stop exercising immediately and call your healthcare provider if you experience these signs during your workouts: sudden or severe abdominal or vaginal pain; any blood or fluid; contractions that go on after you stop exercising; chest pain; shortness of breath; a headache that won't go away; or dizziness. Also, ask yourself: How sore am I after my workouts? Am I really exhausted? Do my joints ache? These factors may help you gauge whether you're pushing yourself a little too hard.

Q / I am a runner. How should I train while I am pregnant?

A: If you were running before pregnancy, you can keep running through the first and second trimesters. But it's not advisable to begin running if you weren't a runner before becoming pregnant. Always discuss your exercise routine with your doctor. If given the green light to run, remember to bring extra water and a cell phone with you, and let someone know where you are running and how long you will be out. In the summer, run in the early morning or evening to avoid excessive heat. And invest in supportive shoes, as pregnancy hormones will affect the arches of your feet. You may need to go up a size, since feet often get larger during pregnancy.

Q / What's one move that will improve my flexibility during pregnancy?

A: You can improve flexibility in a prenatal yoga class or by following an at-home DVD with qualified professionals. During the first trimester, production of the hormone relaxin spikes in your body, loosening joints in the pelvis in preparation for labor. This hormone also makes the rest of the joints in the body lax or unstable, so women who are pregnant must be careful and avoid overstretching. Prenatal yoga moves that work for stretching include gentle upper-body stretches, hip openers and back stretches such as cat and cow poses.

Q / How can I incorporate exercise bands into my pregnancy workout?

A: Try these exercises during your pregnancy:

- Standing arm curl – Stand on the middle of a band, hold the handles and curl your arms.

- Chest press – Wrap a band around a sturdy object and face away from it as you hold a handle in each hand; press forward as if you were doing a push-up.

- Row – Wrap a band around a pole or other sturdy object, face the pole and pull the band toward you, squeezing your upper back.

- Lateral raise – Stand on the middle of a band and raise your arms straight out to the sides.

Your Pre-Pregnancy Gear

- **Maternity workout wear**
  You'll want to stay fit during your pregnancy, and what makes more sense than workout wear that continues to fit you as you grow? Comfortable yoga pants and a maternity workout top will be your key fitness fashions during pregnancy.

- **Yoga mat**
  Just as important as the workout wear is the workout gear. Yoga is a perfect way to work your body and keep it limber during pregnancy, so pick up a yoga mat to keep it cushy on the floor.

- **Tote**
  Not only do you have to carry around your clean snacks; now you'll want to tote your workout gear, extra clothes, a water bottle – and maybe some prenatal vitamins. Give it a personal touch by choosing your favorite color!

105

The number of calories in one banana. It also contains vitamin B6, which helps to alleviate morning sickness.

27mg

THE AMOUNT OF IRON YOU NEED EVERY DAY WHILE PREGNANT. START YOUR DAY WITH A CUP OF PLAIN COOKED OATMEAL – IT HAS 2 MG OF IRON. ADD A TABLESPOON OF TAHINI TO YOUR DAILY DIET AND YOU'LL GET 1.3 MG MORE IRON!

55mg

The amount of vitamin C (which helps keep your skin strong as it stretches) found in one cup of boiled cauliflower.

FIT TIP

"You can never eat too many veggies! As soon as I get home from the grocery store, I wash and cut all my vegetables and toss them into a Ziploc bag. I've often noticed my husband taking advantage of this convenient snack!"

– Julie Bonnett, fitness model

Your Fit Post-Pregnancy FAQ

Q / I need to fit in a quick work-out while my baby sleeps. What's most effective in a short time, yet still safe for after pregnancy?

A: Once you have been approved to work out (generally six to eight weeks postpartum) try this simple full-body workout while baby sleeps:

- **Plié squats** (wide stance) superset with push-ups at three sets of 15 reps each
- **Alternating lunges** (three sets of 12 reps per leg) superset with chair dips (three sets of 15 reps)
- **Regular and reverse abdominal crunches** (three sets of 30 reps each)
- If baby is still asleep, **walk up and down the stairs** for 10 to 15 minutes

Q / I want to improve my upper-body strength so I can carry my baby. What exercises will do this best after my pregnancy?

A: The key to being strong postpartum is continuing to exercise before, during and after pregnancy. Prior to having your baby, do easy upper-body toning exercises – these can include push-ups against the wall, arm curls and arm extensions (dips off a chair). Walking while swinging your arms is another great exercise. Post-delivery, one of the best ways to strengthen your upper body will be carrying your new baby in your arms or in a wrap/baby carrier. If you're looking for more cardio, get out the jogging stroller and go for a walk. As your baby grows and gets heavier, your workout load will become greater and your strength will improve.

Q / What exercises can help me tone up after having a baby without going to the gym?

A: There are many moves you can try without a gym membership. One of the best forms of cardio during or after pregnancy is walking. *Bonus:* A moving stroller can be a great way to calm a crying baby! Great exercises for the lower body include squats as well as stationary and walking lunges. If you have a pair of dumbbells or resistance bands, you can add in curls for your biceps, side raises for your shoulders, overhead extensions for your triceps and chest presses for, you guessed it, your chest.

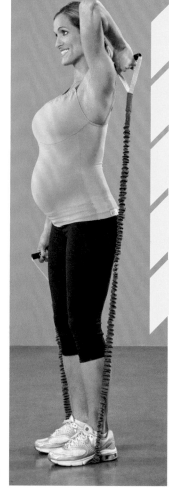

Q / Should I add more abs days to my training routine after having a baby?

A: The key is not adding "more" abs moves, but instead choosing the correct ones. After having a baby, focus on Pilates-type moves that strengthen and pull the transverse muscle in (deepest layer, sometimes referred to as the girdle). A good example is the hover or plank, where there is little movement, just an isometric contraction. You can then gradually add crunches, side crunches and lastly, lower abdominal exercises.

Q / Can you suggest one exercise that will boost my energy after a full day of chasing around a one-year-old?

A: The best post-baby exercise is a walk. Walking elevates the heart rate, exercises all major muscle groups (especially if you hold in your abdominals and swing your arms), has been shown to elevate mood, decreases a mom's overall risk of developing postpartum depression and helps burn off baby weight. If you can't get out of the house, try walking up and down the stairs. Too tired? Find a quiet space and meditate. Meditation will help you refocus for the busy day ahead, recharge your energy and allow your body to be still.

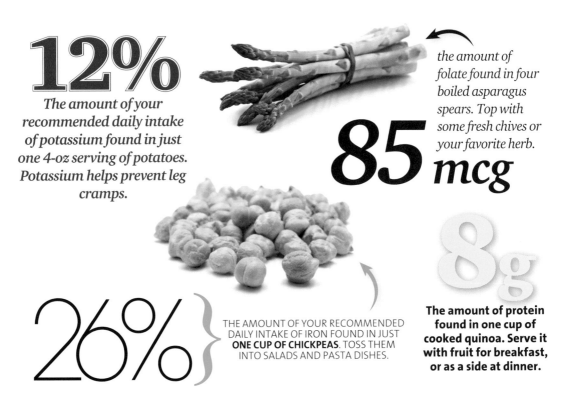

12%

The amount of your recommended daily intake of potassium found in just one 4-oz serving of potatoes. Potassium helps prevent leg cramps.

the amount of folate found in four boiled asparagus spears. Top with some fresh chives or your favorite herb.

85 mcg

8g

The amount of protein found in one cup of cooked quinoa. Serve it with fruit for breakfast, or as a side at dinner.

26%

THE AMOUNT OF YOUR RECOMMENDED DAILY INTAKE OF IRON FOUND IN JUST **ONE CUP OF CHICKPEAS**. TOSS THEM INTO SALADS AND PASTA DISHES.

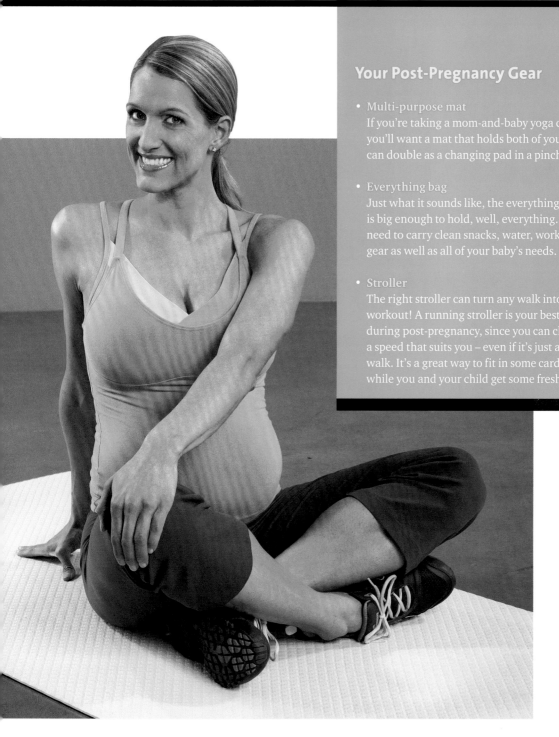

Your Post-Pregnancy Gear

- Multi-purpose mat
  If you're taking a mom-and-baby yoga class, you'll want a mat that holds both of you and can double as a changing pad in a pinch.

- Everything bag
  Just what it sounds like, the everything bag is big enough to hold, well, everything. You'll need to carry clean snacks, water, workout gear as well as all of your baby's needs.

- Stroller
  The right stroller can turn any walk into a workout! A running stroller is your best friend during post-pregnancy, since you can choose a speed that suits you – even if it's just a brisk walk. It's a great way to fit in some cardio while you and your child get some fresh air.

The Oxygen Diet Solution

Success Story

"I feel like I own the gym now!"

BEFORE

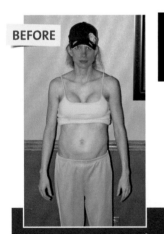

BEFORE: 126 lb
NOW: 126 lb
AGE: 37
HEIGHT: 5'7"
LOCATION: Dubuque, KS
OCCUPATION: Optometrist
FAVORITE EXERCISE:
Back rows

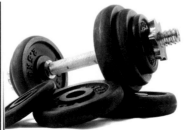

Although the scale never budged, Lynn Howland replaced fat with muscle and gained a fitter, tighter physique. Of all the tricks she's picked up during her journey from "skinny fat" to "muscle mom," she sticks to one rule when pumping iron: "If you don't make an ugly face, you aren't lifting heavy enough."

The Fighter Within

Pushing herself comes naturally to Lynn, whose breast cancer diagnosis back in 2009 propelled her toward fitness and taught her to get tough. "I made the decision that I was in control," she says. She cut back on endless cardio, began to lift heavy ("As much as I could while maintaining proper form!") in a low-rep range, and got serious about building muscle.

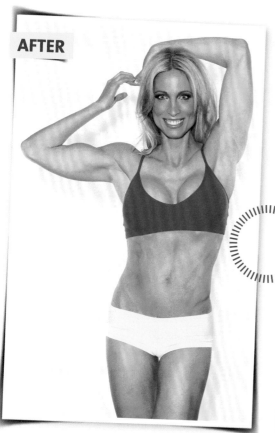

AFTER

"If I want it bad enough, I can achieve it."

Owning It

Cancer free and more confident than ever, Lynn is putting her muscle into shaping up her future with her family. She welcomes new challenges with strength and focus. "I feel like I own the gym now," she says. Most importantly, Lynn now owns total control of her life – and if anybody doesn't like that? Tough.

Power Mornings

Lynn energizes her mornings with a minty mocha protein shake she created to mimic a Starbucks Peppermint Mocha. Lynn's version has a whopping 44 grams of protein! She mixes:

2 scoops chocolate milk-flavored whey protein powder

2 tablespoons peppermint mocha coffee creamer

Cold coffee

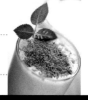

Flexing Mom

As a mom to a seven-year-old daughter and four-year-old son, Lynn couldn't let cancer break her down. She got her children on board, teaching them about the benefits of exercising and eating clean, just as she had learned. Lynn's little ones drink spinach smoothies, which she tells them contain "superhero powers" that will manifest when they turn 18!

Funny Moment

"I was walking through a hotel lobby and a bunch of 10ish-year-old boys waved and yelled, 'Flex!' I flexed my biceps and they ran up to touch it, and then they all started flexing. It made my day!"

Rules of Muscle

According to Lynn, these guidelines are guaranteed to get you a hard body:

1. Do weights before cardio so you're not depleting your energy before you start lifting.

2. Go heavy. "If I can do more than seven reps, I bump up the weight."

3. Perform intervals instead of steady-state cardio. "I go as hard as I can, then recover and repeat. If I get to 20 minutes, it's a rare day!"

4. Immediately after your workout, consume a whey isolate protein shake and a fast-acting carb.

5. Eat! "If you don't eat enough, you won't build muscle."

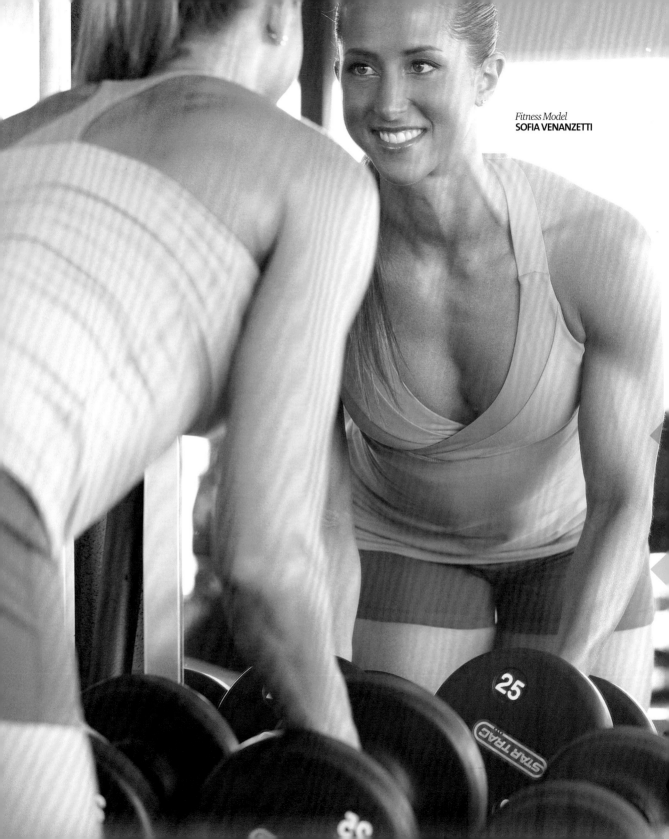

Fitness Model
SOFIA VENANZETTI

Motivation

Everything you need to get off the couch

Motivation – it's the little black dress hiding in your closet, the bikini you haven't worn since your honeymoon and the sexy skinny jeans you keep eyeing at the mall. Or maybe it's that you want to add more energy and excitement to your 9-to-5 lifestyle. Whatever it is for you, we all need something to get ourselves pumped up and driven to achieve our goals, whether we're losing weight to look great or becoming the healthiest that we can be.

There are two types of motivation: intrinsic and extrinsic. Being able to slip on that coveted sexy black dress is the external motivation to lose weight – you want to look good in whatever you wear. But being able to tap into your internal drive will make you more likely to achieve your goals. If you are committed to improving your health and lifestyle, then concentrate on the feeling you get from knowing you are moving toward that goal. This could be the strength and power you feel after working out or the satisfaction of preparing and eating a nutritious meal. Being able to cross off each goal, knowing you've achieved it, is a reward in itself. This is the intrinsic motivation you need to stay dedicated to making a healthy change for yourself, even *after* you manage to fit into that little black dress.

Self-Evaluate

Finding the motivation to create and stick to the *Oxygen* lifestyle is the key to achieving your goals. It all starts with a plan and mapping out the steps needed to take you on your weight-loss journey. The first thing you need to do is a quick self-evaluation.

Take a good look in the mirror. Look at every single part of your body. Make a note of your shoulders, arms, hips, all the way down to your toes. What are your favorite parts? Next, look at what needs improvement. Do you want to tighten that tush or flatten that belly? Write it all down in a journal – including what you love about yourself – to help you decide what your health and fitness goals will be. Once you've written everything down you can move on to the next step: writing out your goals and planning your weight-loss journey!

Just remember, a lifestyle change involves revamping the way you think about yourself. You are the change you've been waiting for, and staying positive during your weight-loss journey will help fuel your motivation. Believe in yourself and know that you will achieve your goals and be the best you can be. Take 10 minutes each morning to look in the mirror and say "I CAN and WILL work toward achieving a fit body!" Think back to a time when you did accomplish something you worked hard for – whether it was buying your first house or finishing a college course; remember that feeling of satisfaction and excitement. Know that you can be successful again and again!

Setting Goals

It's never too early or too late to set goals and create a plan to achieve those goals. It's as easy as grabbing a journal and starting to write. First, think about what you need in order to be successful. Are you a morning person? Can you wake up an hour early each morning to work out? Do you need to join a gym to get moving or will you find it more comfortable to exercise in your own home (and will you actually do it)? Do you need a friend to help you stay motivated? Questions like these will help you create a success plan that is sure to produce results. And make sure you answer honestly. If the truth is that you will not motivate yourself to work out at home because you have too many distractions, then it does you no good to pretend you will.

Now the most important part: setting, writing down and committing to your goals. You want to think long term and short term, and make sure they are realistic and attainable. You know you're not going to run a half-marathon by next week, so don't make that your goal. Unless you are vastly overweight, you won't lose 10 pounds by next week either. You can set small weekly goals for yourself – maybe you can jog/walk one mile by next week, for example – and then set longer-term goals such as running a half- or even a full marathon in 12 months. Pacing yourself and knowing your limits will allow you to achieve each goal, one after the other. And those small goals all bring you to your large goal in the long run. Since larger goals can seem too intimidating and the results too far off, setting smaller ones in between will let you celebrate wins more often.

Make sure you figure out which type of training methods and eating plans you need to accomplish your goals. Plan where you want your health and physique to be within the next six months to a year. The next step is to do your research. There are many different myths about working out and proper supplementation, so it's best to speak to a personal trainer or other health and fitness expert and read health and fitness books (like this one) and magazines such as *Oxygen*. Also, keep a journal to log your progress and your day-to-day habits. Take measurements of your body regularly, but not too often, to gauge if you're getting closer to your goals. If you're not getting the results you had hoped for and expected, then review your workouts – are you working hard enough, for example? – and your diet. Are you eating too many meals or snacks that are not part of your chosen diet? Are your portions too large? Take this time to write your goals in a journal or in the Goal Setting section starting on p. 282.

Once you've written down all your goals, post them somewhere you'll see them every day. Whether you write them on a calendar at work or tape them to your bathroom mirror, seeing them every day will keep you inspired and remind you to keep your head in the game. You can even create an inspiration board by posting up pictures of your role models, your goals, inspirational quotes or pictures of a healthier you! Not only is it a fun and inspiring activity, it's a great way to visualize the life you want to achieve.

Make sure you take some time at the beginning of each week to plan out how you will accomplish your goals. Get rid of all the junk food in your kitchen and fill it with healthy staples to prevent you from sabotaging your weight-loss goals. Plan each workout session, whether you do it at home as soon as you get up, during your lunch hour or in the evening at the gym. Decide in advance what you're going to do during your workout so you don't waste time. You can

even ask a friend to join you or hire a personal trainer to make you more accountable. Write your exercise and meal times down in ink and commit 100 percent to staying on schedule – and you will succeed! As *Oxygen*'s late founder Robert Kennedy said in his book *Bull's Eye*, "Don't put a hold on your decision to act. Don't postpone joy."

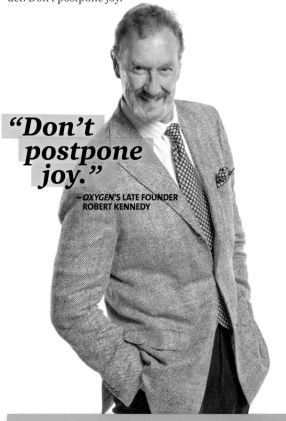

"Don't postpone joy."

— OXYGEN'S LATE FOUNDER
ROBERT KENNEDY

FIT TIP

"I use a dry erase board to plot out my travel plans, social events and competitions for the month. This allows me to plan my fitness around all of life's other obligations, and ensure I'm getting all of my training in."

– *Natalie Waples, fitness model*

SMART GOAL SETTING: YOUR KEY TO SUCCESS

THIS IS IT. You're armed with a pen and a journal. All you need to do is write down the words that will pave the way to your success. When you're writing down your short-term and long-term goals, keep the SMART acronym in mind:

S **SPECIFIC** – Make sure you choose a goal that is specific. As opposed to writing: "I want to lose weight," for example, you should set specific targets, such as "I want to lose 20 pounds" or "I want to do 200 push-ups." This will help you determine your plan of action. You can lose 20 pounds, for example, by committing to the Basic *Oxygen* Diet meal plan and an exercise regimen.

M **MEASURABLE** – How are you going to measure the progress you're making toward your goal? How many goals have you written and is it possible to achieve them all? Set up an outline of how you're going to stay on track and reach your targets in the time you've set aside to achieve them. How will you know you have accomplished your goals? Whether it's seeing the scale drop by 20 pounds or the muscle definition appearing, make sure you make note of each small change to help you stay on target.

A **ATTAINABLE** – Make sure you write down goals you know you can achieve. Losing 20 pounds in three months is definitely possible. However, if you want to lose 20 pounds in one month or do a set of 200 push-ups right off the bat, then you should probably rethink your strategy. Always ask yourself, are these goals attainable in the amount of time given?

R **REALISTIC** – You know it's more likely that you'll do a set of 10 or 20 push-ups than 200. Keep it real and know what your strengths and weaknesses are. Although it may be possible for you, as a beginner, to achieve a fitness model physique in a year's time, it isn't likely you'll hit the front cover of *Oxygen* magazine in the same time. If that is your goal, you may end up disappointed. Look at your options and figure out where your health and fitness levels are when you first start out. This will provide a basis for you to set realistic goals.

T **TIMELY** – How much time will it take for you to lose those 20 pounds? You know healthy and permanent weight loss doesn't happen overnight, much as you may wish otherwise. If your goal is to lose 20 pounds in one month and you end up losing 10 pounds, you will feel like a failure instead of the success you are. Give yourself enough time to achieve your goals.

FIT TIP

"My main motivator is to be a role model for my daughter and have the energy to be an active mother. I owe my daughter the best habits I can instill in her. She motivates me to be a better and healthier person."

– Kim Dolan Leto, fitness model

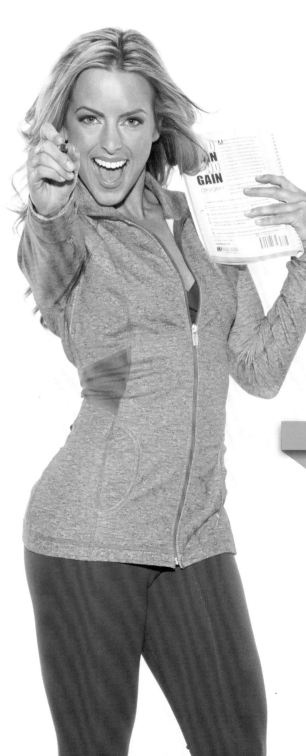

Now, turn to p. 282 and write down your personal data, measurements and goals. Start with your long-term goal. Then figure out what you need to do on a daily and weekly basis to get there.

Fitness Model
LINDSAY MESSINA

FIT TIP

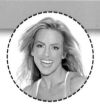

"As long as you're completely focused on your goals, and you know what you really want, then you will find it easier to follow your weight-loss plan – even on weekends!"

– Lindsay Messina, fitness model

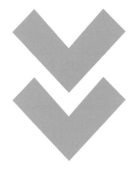

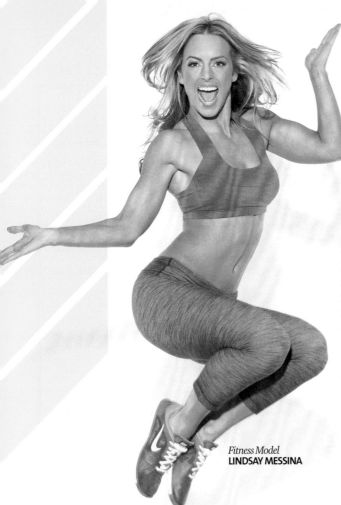

Fitness Model
LINDSAY MESSINA

As a fitness celebrity, Lindsay hears a lot of excuses. People fall off the health and fitness wagon for many reasons, such as traveling for work, an illness, feeling too tired to hit the gym or not having the time to make healthy meals. However, these are just excuses to Lindsay. Now is the time to ditch those excuses and take your life back! Here are the top three excuses she hears and her tips on how to beat them.

Excuse: When I was your age, I could work out the way you do, but now I'm too old. I used to be able to do anything.

LINDSAY SAYS: Actually, many women twice my age have better bodies than I do, and seem to be able to fit working out and eating right into their schedule. They structure their day-to-day lives in order to care for their families and maintain their work schedule. Time is minimal, and that makes them motivated to fit their "me time" in so they can feel good. A woman who works out and eats right feels happier, which affects the way she handles her husband and kids. I find that fit, older women tend to work out harder and structure their time better because it makes them feel great all the way around.

LINDSAY'S SOLUTION: Take one day to write out your schedule for the week and make sure to take at least an hour each day to focus on yourself. Whether that means cooking your healthy meals for the week or heading to the gym, it is definitely possible to stick to the *Oxygen* lifestyle at any age!

No Excuses!

Fitness star and *Oxygen Diet Solution* cover girl Lindsay Messina shares her secrets for getting (and staying!) motivated.

Sticking to your weight-loss plan and a healthy lifestyle can be tricky when you're taking care of a family, working full time, taking part in social activities and dealing with whatever else life throws your way. So how does our cover model Lindsay Messina stay fit while juggling her busy schedule? It's all about planning ahead and preparing yourself for a variety of situations. For Lindsay, it comes down to how badly you want to lose those pounds, build muscle or look and feel your best.

Excuse: I work full time and I can't seem to fit working out and cooking healthy meals into my schedule.

LINDSAY SAYS: There are always options to make your schedule work for you. You can wake up a little bit earlier and bring your work clothes to the gym with you. Once you do this for two weeks or so, your body will get used to waking up early and going to the gym. Or you can work out during your lunch hour, take some extra time getting home from work, or work out instead of watching TV in the evening. The key is getting into the habit of doing it, since your body will actually crave it. Eventually you'll find that if you miss your gym date, you won't feel good throughout the day. That's the state you want to achieve.

LINDSAY'S SOLUTION: Wake up at least 45 minutes early and get to the gym at least three times per week, which will keep you amped up throughout your day. If you're not a morning person, pack your gym clothes, put them in your car and train at lunch or drive straight to the gym after work to spend at least an hour working out. It's better to hit the gym before you head home and make dinner – nine times out of 10 you may not talk yourself into heading back out.

Excuse: It's easier for me to stick to a schedule during the week. On the weekend I seem to go off the rails!

LINDSAY SAYS: As long as you're completely focused on your goals, and you know what you really want, then you will find it easier to follow your weight-loss plan – even on weekends! When someone wants to change her lifestyle badly enough, anything is possible. Don't beat yourself up if you can't stay clean all seven days. In fact, it should be easier for you to make those healthier food choices on the weekend because you tend to have more free time for preparation. And remember you need to incorporate one rest day in between your workouts.

LINDSAY'S SOLUTION: If you, your partner or kids crave burgers on the weekend, you don't need to serve them fatty ground beef. Instead, make lean meat burgers or bean burgers, grill them and instead of hamburger buns you can use whole wheat bread or English muffins. Instead of greasy fries, you can bake some sweet potato fries. Get your kids to help you season the fries with sea salt and help you cook. Enlist your family's help and you can have fun keeping it clean on the weekends.

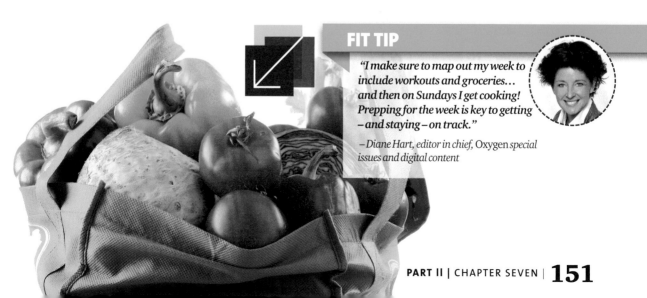

FIT TIP

"I make sure to map out my week to include workouts and groceries… and then on Sundays I get cooking! Prepping for the week is key to getting – and staying – on track."

– *Diane Hart, editor in chief,* Oxygen *special issues and digital content*

Lindsay's Top Tips for Social Situations

When you know you've got a dinner date or you're spending your Friday night with the girls, chances are drinks and calorie-laden foods will be involved. Being aware of this is the first step to avoid straying from your plan to lose fat or build muscle. Here are Lindsay's tricks for staying on track at social gatherings:

- **If you do decide to have alcohol,** avoid the sugary, fruity drinks and stick to the clear ones. Go for wine or a wine spritzer instead of those multi-colored martinis and keep it to a minimum. Also, drink water along with your alcoholic beverage.

- **Choose between a drink and a dessert** instead of having both, to reduce your caloric intake.

- **Stay away from starchy and fried foods** when you eat at restaurants.

- **Remember, don't be hard on yourself** if you occasionally indulge. Simply jump back on your weight-loss journey the next day!

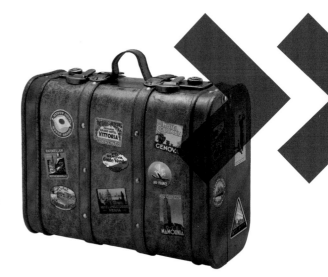

Lindsay's Travel Tips

Part of being a fitness model involves traveling, so Lindsay always has a plan to keep her diet and exercise on track. If you're going to be traveling a lot, know that your gym regimen isn't going to be the same as it is at home, and plan accordingly. Here are some tricks to keep in mind:

- **Make time for at least 20 minutes of cardio** to kick up your metabolism, especially if you know you'll be consuming more calories. Try skipping rope, going for a jog, taking a walk or even walking up and down the hotel stairs.

- **Pack dry foods such as unsalted** almonds, protein powder and oatmeal. Pre-plan your meals and, if possible, bring a cooler filled with cooked lean meat and raw veggies to make sure you're getting solid meals throughout your day. You can also map out any grocery stores that will be near to where you are staying.

- **Remember, temporarily you may not** be progressing with your goals but following these tips will help sustain you and allow you to feel better when your schedule isn't on point.

For more on staying fit while traveling, see the Fit Travels section on p. 156.

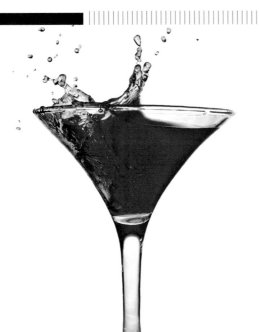

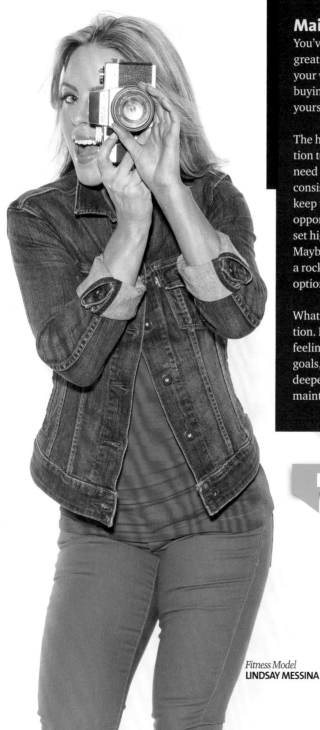

Maintenance: Staying the Course

You've done it – you've reached your goals, you feel great and you're looking your best. First, celebrate your win by donning your little black dress or finally buying those sexy skinny jeans at the mall. Reward yourself; you deserve it!

The hard part is over, and now finding the motivation to maintain your health is strong. But you still need to plan, update your goals and maintain a consistent schedule of training and eating right to keep the body you've always wanted. Here's the opportunity for you to mix up your workout routine, set higher goals and step out of your comfort zone. Maybe you want to enter a fitness competition, gain a rock-hard six-pack or do a one-arm pull up. Your options are endless!

What helps to sustain your success is inner motivation. Remember, it is the intrinsic desire, or the feeling and power you get from accomplishing your goals, that allows you to stay on track. Pinpointing a deeper drive to live a healthy lifestyle will help you maintain the change you've worked so hard for.

FIT TIP

"Recently, when I found my motivation lagging, I turned to my husband for some gentle encouragement. I told him when the alarm goes off at 5:30 and I'm procrastinating on getting out of bed, I need him to 'lovingly' tell me it's time to get up and get to the gym. Of course, I get grumpy when he does it, but it works like a charm."

– *Stacy Rinella, editor in chief*

Fitness Model
LINDSAY MESSINA

LINDSAY'S TOP 3 MOTIVATORS FOR MAINTENANCE

1 / Health:

"My family has struggled with obesity, yo-yo diet-ing, diabetes and high cholesterol. So for me, it's just knowing that I don't want to live that lifestyle. I don't want to live my life taking blood pressure medica-tion or insulin. Watching my blood sugar levels or taking cholesterol pills in the morning in order to maintain the status quo is not the way of life for me. We are in control of our health."

tip *Keeping a clean diet of whole grains, fruits, vegetables and lean proteins will amp up your immune system and keep you strong. Pair clean eating with a regular workout schedule or active lifestyle, and you will be well on your way to good health.*

2 / Physique:

"I really love a beautiful physique that is tight and has perfect muscular tone. That's what makes me tick. When I see other fitness athletes in magazines with rock-hard abs, they inspire me. I read up on their workouts and learn. They probably read up on mine too, so it's a full circle of people who inspire each other. When I see other athletes raising the bar, it makes me want to do the same."

tip *Read up on your favorite fitness experts like Lindsay in Oxygen magazine. Find out what the pros are eating and how they're changing up their workout routines. Keeping things interesting is a good way to help you maintain your healthy lifestyle.*

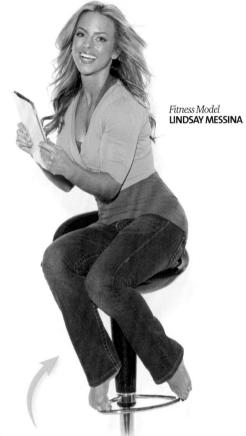

Fitness Model
LINDSAY MESSINA

3 / Helping others:

"Getting comments on Facebook and receiving emails from people who have changed their lives by following my workouts or diet is a wonderful feeling. I'm helping others live a healthy lifestyle by writing my column or posting my recipes online. That really drives me on an everyday basis."

tip *Start a blog or keep track of your progress on your Facebook or Twitter accounts. Invite your friends over for a healthy dinner party, or for a picnic at the end of a hike. You never know which of your friends will be inspired to join your healthy way of living.*

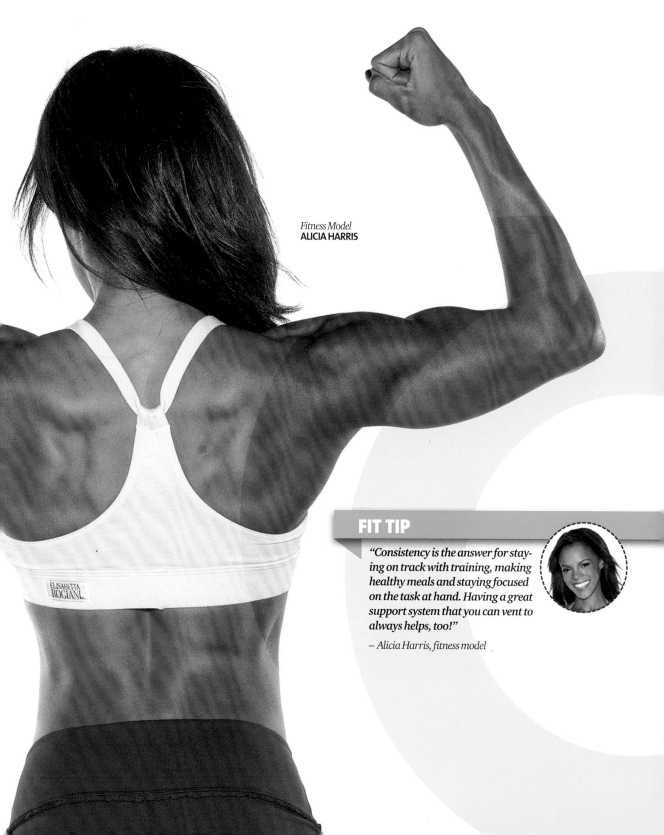

Fitness Model
ALICIA HARRIS

Fit Travels

6 WAYS TO STAY FIT WHILE TRAVELING

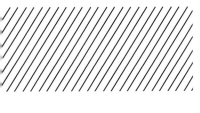

You're committed to living the *Oxygen* lifestyle and you're on your way to achieving your health and fitness goals. But suddenly your boss wants you to go on a five-day business trip. How can you eat clean and exercise with a jam-packed traveling schedule and when you're living out of a hotel room?

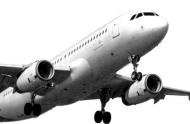

Don't panic! It is possible to stick to your healthy living plan, whether you're on a business trip, a vacation or backpacking for a year – it just takes a little planning and foresight. Here are six nutrition and exercise tips to help you avoid weight gain while away from home.

1 / Pack food for the trip.

Pack snacks in your carry-on bag to avoid bland and unhealthy plane food. Opt for pre-cooked sliced chicken, unsalted nuts, sliced veggies, fruits with a peel and whole-grain bread slices or crispbreads. Make sure you stick to water and avoid sugary drinks and alcohol. In your luggage, you can bring pre-measured oatmeal separated into baggies, natural nut butter, protein powder and a water bottle. You can also request a fridge, microwave and coffee maker for your hotel room.

2 / Head to the grocery store.

When you arrive, you can buy some pre-grilled rotisserie chicken, apples, berries, pre-sliced vegetables, more unsalted nuts and bottled water to store in your hotel fridge.

FIT TIP

"I always carry a water bottle and protein bar in my purse. I'm very forgetful! Packing them first thing in the morning keeps me hydrated and on track to eat well when in a crunch."

– Melissa Hall, fitness model

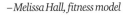

3/ Eating out? Choose wisely.

It's inevitable – you will hit up local restaurants or maybe even fast food joints while you're traveling. But as long as you plan ahead, you can be ready for anything! Stick to dishes that are baked or grilled, order extra steamed vegetables and avoid anything cooked with butter and added salt. Ask for sauces on the side, or avoid them altogether. Order water, skip the booze and leave before you order a double fudge chocolate cake for dessert. Also, remember to watch your portions – you can always take a doggy bag to save for lunch the next day!

4/ Avoid cabs and take a walk instead.

Walking to your business conference or to sightsee around the city is a great way to stay active. Not only does this save money and burn calories, you can also take in more of the culture around you. Wear comfortable shoes (or carry flip-flops in your purse if you need to wear heels to a meeting or social event) and be sure to ask the front desk staff if the area is safe to walk in!

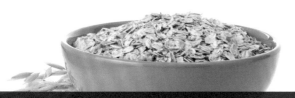

ON-THE-GO OATMEAL

½ cup whole oats	Mix all ingredients together and pour into a resealable bag to take with you wherever you go. Simply pour the mixture into a container, add hot water, mix and enjoy your clean breakfast!
2 tbsp ground flaxseed	
1 scoop protein powder	
A scant handful of unsweetened dried fruit	
Pinch cinnamon	

5/ Kick-start your day with exercise.

If your schedule is packed with tours and museum visits or meetings and dinners, plan to work out as soon as you get up in the morning. This way you can shower and get ready to conquer the rest of your day, feeling great knowing that your workout is done.

6/ Have a game plan.

Finding a hotel with a gym is the best way to squeeze in a sweat session, and luckily most hotels – even the inexpensive ones – do have gyms these days. But no need to worry if your hotel doesn't have a gym. The trick is to pack portable equipment, such as a resistance band to work those muscles and a jump rope for cardio. It's fun, fast and you'll feel the burn! You can bring some workout routines with you as well, such as the On-the-Go Resistance Band Workout on the following pages. You can work out right in your hotel room, even in your pajamas (or your birthday suit, for that matter)! No need to worry about gym clothes or keeping your hair back. You can also do a hotel room circuit of bodyweight exercises: pushups, lunges and squats are great options. A bonus: adapting your workout while on the road will allow you to stimulate different muscles. If your workouts have been getting stale, you may even find some renewed muscle action!

Your On-the-Go Resistance Band Workout

Resistance bands are easy to carry around, and you can complete these exercises right in your hotel room. Do the following routine two or three times, resting for one to two minutes between circuits. Complete 10–20 reps per set.

TOOLS FOR TRAVEL:

- Resistance band
- Jump rope
- Water bottle

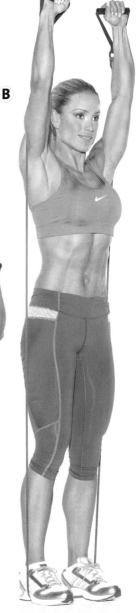

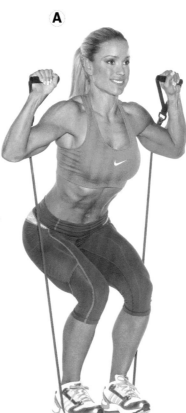

1// *Squat and Press*

TARGET MUSCLES:
QUADRICEPS, GLUTES, FRONT AND MIDDLE DELTOIDS (SHOULDERS)

SET UP/ Stand in the center of the band with feet hip-width apart. Hold band handles above shoulder height, palms in front and facing away from you.

ACTION/ Squat until your thighs are parallel to the floor **[A]**. Press through your heels to stand back up. Drive the band handles toward the ceiling as you reach full extension **[B]**. Reverse the move and return to starting position.

2// Balancing Triceps Extension

TARGET MUSCLES:
TRICEPS, TRANSVERSE ABDOMINIS

SET UP/ Stand on one end of the band with your right foot and hold the other end in your right hand. Lift your elbow so it points toward the ceiling and drop your hand beneath your head **[A]**. Place your left hand on your waist and lift your left knee to hip height in front of you.

ACTION/ Straighten your right arm toward the ceiling, keeping your upper arm close to your ear and your core tight **[B]**. Pause at full extension then slowly lower to starting position. Complete all reps on right side then switch to left.

3// Lunge with a Curl

TARGET MUSCLES:
QUADRICEPS, GLUTES, BICEPS

SET UP/ Step on center of the band with your right foot. Hold handles at your sides, arms in close to your body, palms forward. Take a big step back with your left foot.

ACTION/ Keeping your upper arms stationary, curl handles toward your shoulders **[A]**. Hold this position as you lower your body into a lunge **[B]**. Pause, then press through right heel to stand. Slowly lower handles back to sides. Complete all reps on right leg before switching to left.

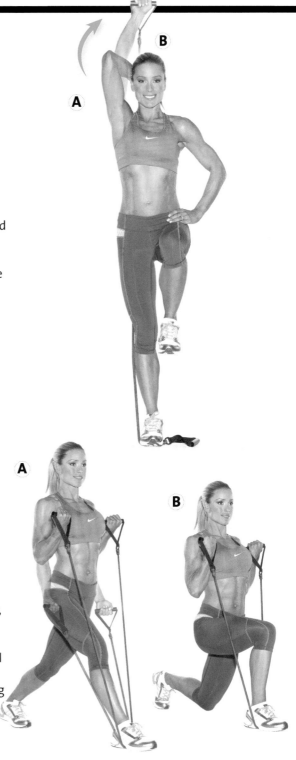

4// *Deadlift with Row*

TARGET MUSCLES:
HAMSTRINGS, GLUTES, BACK, REAR DELTOIDS
(SHOULDERS)

SET UP/ Knot a loop in the band and stand on
the band with both feet. Hold the handles in
front of your thighs with palms facing inward.

ACTION/ Fold forward from your hips, with
knees slightly bent, until your torso makes a
45-degree angle to perpendicular **[A]**. Pull both
handles toward your rib cage, squeezing your
shoulder blades together while keeping arms
close to your sides **[B]**. Pause, then lower hands
and use hamstrings and glutes to raise body
back to starting position. Repeat.

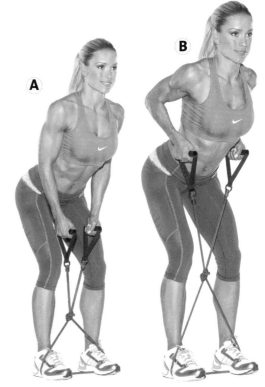

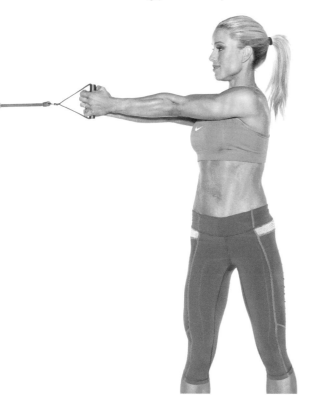

5// *Torso Rotation*

TARGET MUSCLES:
OBLIQUES, TRANSVERSE ABDOMINIS, REAR AND
MIDDLE DELTOIDS, CHEST, UPPER BACK

SET UP/ Anchor a band at shoulder height to a
stationary object or wrap around the doorknob
on the opposite side of a door and shut firmly.
Stand sideways to the anchor, feet shoulder-
width apart for stability. Grasp handle with
straight arms at chest height, and rotate torso
and shoulders away from the anchor, stretching
the band as you pull it across your body to face
the opposite direction. Slowly uncoil and return
to starting position. Complete all reps on one
side then switch to other side.

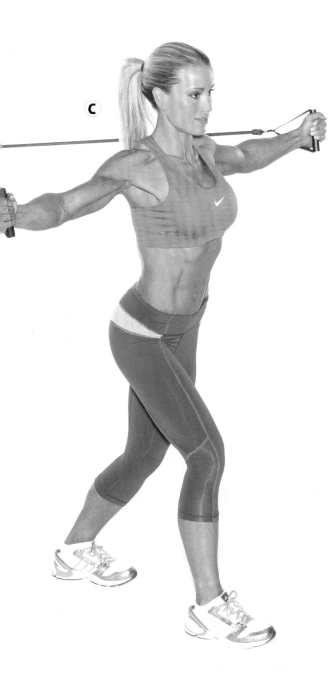

C

6// *Chest Press and Flye*

TARGET MUSCLES:
CHEST, FRONT DELTOIDS (SHOULDERS)

SET UP/ Anchor the center of the band to a stationary object or wrap around doorknob on the opposite side of a door and shut firmly. Facing away from the anchor, hold handles at shoulder height and take a large step forward with one foot. Extend arms parallel to the ground, palms facing downward **[A]**.

ACTION/ Bend elbows to bring your hands back toward your shoulders **[B]**. Smoothly reverse the move, pressing handles to an extended position **[A]**. Turn your palms inward, bend your elbows slightly and open your arms wide until your elbows come in line with your torso **[C]**. Slowly reverse the move to bring the handles back to starting position **[A]**. Continue, alternating presses and flyes.

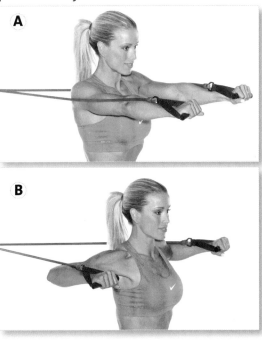

A

B

Tips from Tosca's Trainer

RITA CATOLINO SHARES HER SECRETS FOR SUCCESS

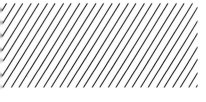

Rita Catolino never thought she'd get to know, much less train, bestselling author and columnist Tosca Reno. But the day she picked up *The Eat-Clean Diet® Cookbook* was also the day she made up her mind to take a different path. "That book changed my life," says the now slim and toned Rita, who coached Tosca right into the number-one spot in the Bikini Grand Masters category at the Kitchener-Waterloo Oktoberfest Classic in 2012. Motivated by Tosca's book, Rita made clean eating a part of every day, filling her own cooler with fresh veggies and grilled chicken, and bringing it with her to the gym. She even became an eat-clean advocate, walking the walk with clients, friends and family.

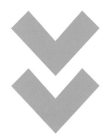

"Because I know where I've come from, I don't ever want to be there again."

RITA CATOLINO,
PERSONAL TRAINER
BEFORE: 160 lb
NOW: 132 lb
AGE: 32
HEIGHT: 5'7"
LOCATION: London, Ontario, Canada
LOST: 15% body fat, 28lb

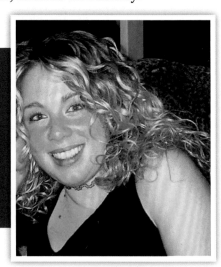

This wasn't always the case with the self-confessed pasta lover. In fact, rewind a few years when the fun-loving Rita was a much different person – she weighed about 30 pounds more than she does today, and her body fat percentage hovered in the 30-percent range. One day, she looked into her closet and faced a harsh truth: she couldn't fit into any of her clothes. She recalls too clearly the realization that her weight was slowly climbing, and all she did was continue to eat while working hard in school.

Growing up with strict Italian parents, she was always in a protected environment – her parents even picked her up every day after her college classes. Though she can't imagine life without her workouts today, they weren't part of her life back then. But a trip to Spain, where she walked everywhere and ate healthier, started to have its effect, and when she returned to Canada one year later after meeting the love of her life, husband Dario, she began to understand the value of a changed lifestyle.

Tosca's book gave her a much-needed plan she could map out. It also instilled in her the confidence she needed to get on stage. Venturing into competitions, Rita has competed in 11 contests to date. "Because I know where I've come from, I don't ever want to be there again," says Rita of her determination to never go back to her former lifestyle.

Rita took up the challenge of total-body change with all the tenacity, determination and work ethic that she inherited from her parents – her father arrived in the country with only a battered suitcase, but what he had was a tremendous capacity for hard work. "He worked every day of his life for 37 years and never missed a day of work," she says.

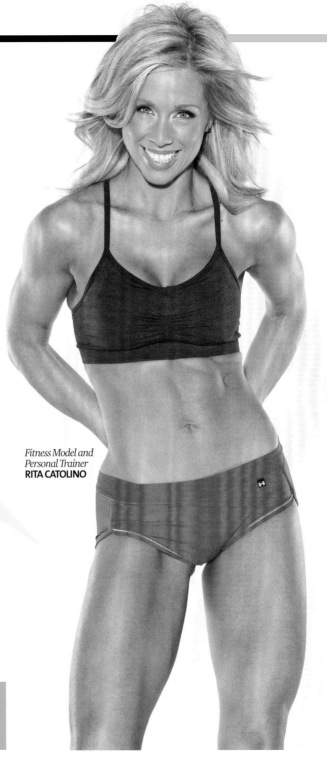

Fitness Model and Personal Trainer
RITA CATOLINO

Her mother tried every diet without success and constantly battled a weight problem. But when Rita's now five-year-old daughter, Ariana, was born, Rita recalls thinking this was her opportunity to break the cycle of perpetual yo-yo dieting that rarely results in sustainable change.

"I was determined to do it," she says.

Today, Rita keeps busy training clients, traveling and entertaining. Despite the large part that training plays in her life, she still enjoys gathering in her home with family and friends, and bonding over a delicious meal.

"I love to cook – you need to enjoy your food!" says Rita.

What you don't need to do, she says, is continue to make excuses for not being the person you can be. "You must envision what you want and then set the goals that will get you there – and follow through!" Rita notes that it may not happen overnight, but if you seek sustainable change, you will have to work for it. She tries to instill in her clients a love of the journey rather than the end result. For Rita, it's far better to immerse yourself in the challenge and enjoy your experiences along the way.

RITA'S TOP TIP:

"Stick to a plan that speaks to you, not anyone else."

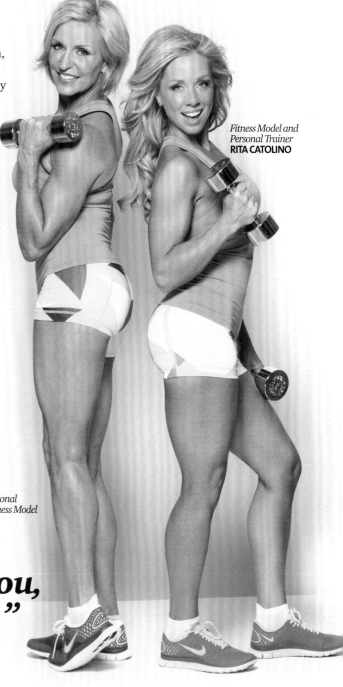

Fitness Model and Personal Trainer
RITA CATOLINO

Author, Motivational Speaker and Fitness Model
TOSCA RENO

RITA'S "CLEAN" TORTILLA DE PATATAS ESPAÑOLA

Makes 4–6 servings

3 medium-sized sweet potatoes, chopped

2 medium onions, diced

3 eggs

7 egg whites

2 tbsp olive oil

Sea salt and pepper, to taste

Pimentón (a smoky Spanish spice), optional

1. In a pot, boil potatoes for 10 to 15 minutes.

2. Heat oil over medium heat in a nonstick pan. Sauté onions until translucent. Add potatoes, stirring occasionally to prevent sticking, until they are a little golden and cooked all the way through. Add a dash of salt and pepper, or pimentón.

3. Meanwhile, in a bowl, lightly beat eggs and egg whites with a fork.

4. When potato mixture is cooked, add to bowl with eggs. Mix with a wooden spoon. Add the mixture back to the pan. Let mixture sit to cook through, and for edges to solidify. Use a large plate to flip and cook on the other side, until slightly golden brown. Remove and serve warm.

RITA'S TOP TIP:

"Ditch excuses. You're not allowing yourself to be the optimal person you can be. Excuses are just excuses."

Rita's Eat-Clean Tips & Tricks

Rita Catolino loves to cook – and it shows. Here are her top tips for keeping your diet clean, easy and delicious!

"I have 15 to 20 almonds in mini Ziploc bags 'hidden' in various places: glove compartment, gym bag, every purse and my desk at work. That way I always have something to munch on between meals, without overdoing it and eating the whole bag!"

"I hard boil 12 eggs every Sunday and have them peeled and ready to go for an easy snack on the go – protein and fat in one perfect package given to us by nature."

"Switch up your protein choices to keep your body guessing. Try bison burgers, lamb, rabbit, mussels – all great sources of lean protein!"

"When I'm looking to lean out for an upcoming show or shoot, I rely on fresh seafood as protein sources: shrimp, salmon, tilapia, cod, sole. They keep me full and are easier to digest than heavier meats."

"Make sure to change your flavor profile when using the same protein choices so that you don't get bored. Try salmon with ginger or capers, or lemon and dill, or coriander and paprika! New dish every time!"

The **oxygen** *Diet Solution* Success *Story*

IN JUST SIX MONTHS,
JENNA DUNHAM
DROPPED 70 POUNDS –
AND HER "FAT PANTS."

"I really wanted to be a fit mom!"

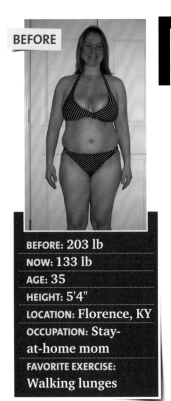

BEFORE

BEFORE: 203 lb

NOW: 133 lb

AGE: 35

HEIGHT: 5'4"

LOCATION: Florence, KY

OCCUPATION: Stay-at-home mom

FAVORITE EXERCISE: Walking lunges

Judging by the timid smile in her "After" picture, you might not take Jenna Dunham for the type of woman who rocks out to Metallica in the weight room. Then again, you might not take her for someone who once found herself in size XL maternity pants. But it's her abs that give away Jenna's proudest fit secret: a mother of three, she's worked her butt off to attain them.

Fit Words

After her third pregnancy, Jenna found motivation in an unlikely place: the "F" word. "I was 203 pounds and 'frumpy,'" she says. Jenna felt discouraged, but relied on a personal mantra to get back into the gym. "I can do anything for one minute," she told herself before stepping on the treadmill or walking over to the weights area. Soon, she was up to sprints and advanced strength-training circuits.

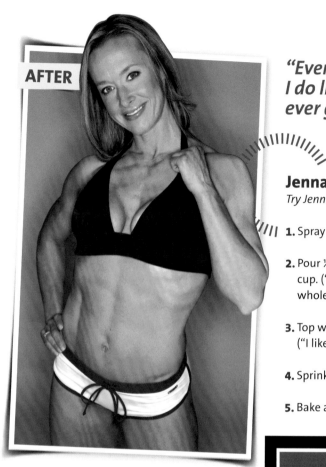

AFTER

> *"Everything I do in the gym, I do like it's the last time I'll ever get to do it."*

Jenna's Protein On the Go
Try Jenna's abs-friendly protein cups:

1. Spray a muffin tin with nonstick cooking spray.

2. Pour ¼ cup egg whites into each muffin cup. ("You can also crack one whole egg into each cup!")

3. Top with chopped veggies ("I like red peppers and mushrooms.").

4. Sprinkle with fat-free feta cheese.

5. Bake at 375°F until whites are firm.

Muscle Mom

Metal music aside, a desire to become a fit mom – not just a skinny one – was Jenna's driving force. Within six months, she lost 70 pounds, reduced her body fat from 31 to 17 percent, and increased her strength. As for those abs, she stuck with a clean diet, returned to Pilates and fell in love with circuit training. With a stronger body and mind, she became a happier mom.

In her closet, Jenna keeps the XL maternity pants ("the largest pair of pants I've ever worn!") to remind her of how far she's come. Now, she's swapped them out for a pair of slim skinny jeans that show off her shapely glutes and toned quads. So much for being frumpy.

Bouncing Back

"Some women make it look so easy to get back into shape after having a baby," says Jenna, "but it takes a ton of hard work!" Below, her top three tips for bouncing back:

1. Rely on a good support network of friends and family (Jenna's husband even made a shirt with her face on it!).

2. Try new workout classes and routines.

3. Write down your goals for the day/week/month.

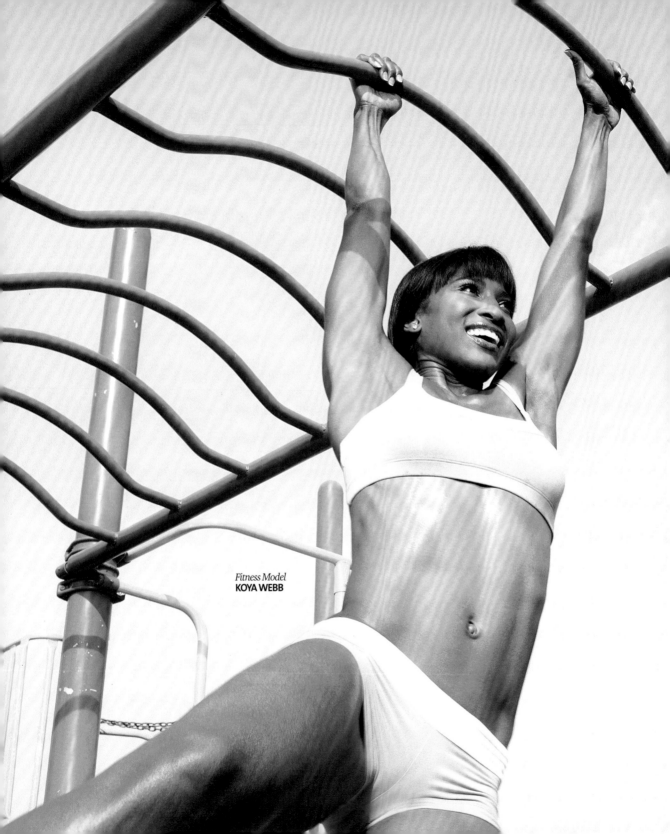

Fitness Model
KOYA WEBB

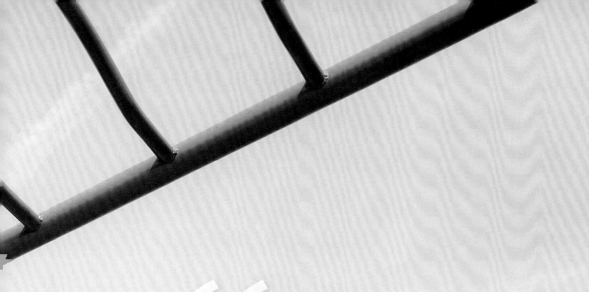

"Success does not come from perfection; it comes from consistently *moving in the right direction.***"**

— TOSCA RENO,
AUTHOR, MOTIVATIONAL
SPEAKER AND FITNESS MODEL

PART III

FOOD AND SUPPLEMENTS

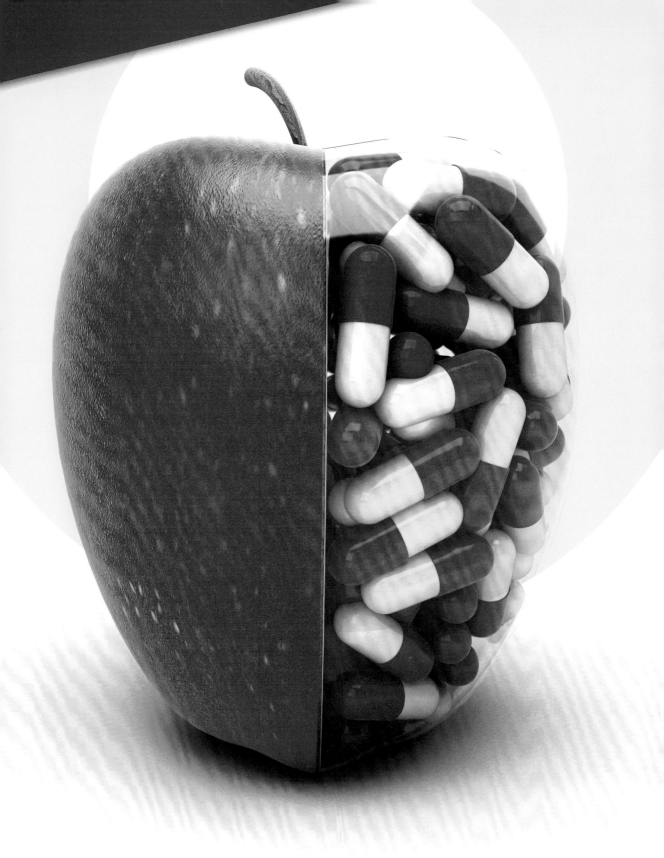

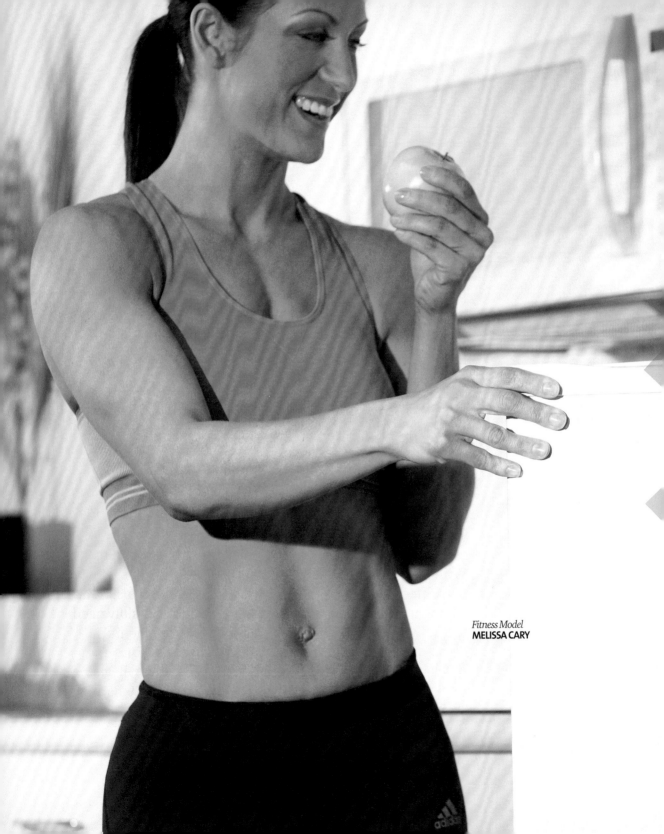

Fitness Model
MELISSA CARY

All About Food

Fuel up for a great body!

With Susan Kleiner's detailed meal plans to guide you through every bite on the way to achieving your goals, right now you might be thinking, "What else could I possibly need to know about food?" Well, how about the fundamentals of eating clean courtesy of Tosca Reno? Or Jamie Eason's take on calorie counting? This section of the book will also help you troubleshoot a variety of diet dilemmas, including nighttime cravings and breakfast blunders, and that will definitely put you on the fast track to success!

The Eat-Clean Commandments

The Eat-Clean Diet® queen and *Oxy* gal extraordinaire Tosca Reno shares her 10 simple rules for a lifetime of healthy eating.

1 / Say no to sugar.

It's been called the "arch enemy of health" – and with good reason! Sugar has been linked to a variety of diseases and health issues, including immune suppression, inflammation, diabetes, liver fatigue and even some cancers.

2 / Get to know this power couple: LP + CC.

You'll notice that all of the meal plans in this book ensure you will be eating a combination of lean protein (chicken, salmon, beans, etc.) and complex carbohydrates (whole grains, fresh fruits and veggies) at each meal. This power couple is your key to metabolism- and health-boosting results.

3 / Eat five or six small meals a day.

This keeps your metabolism stimulated while preventing you from going hungry and feeling deprived – just make sure these meals contain LP + CC and are comprised of clean (i.e., natural and non-processed) foods.

4 / Don't skip meals – especially breakfast.

Skipping meals not only leads to bingeing, but also means you've effectively geared down your metabolism and lost an opportunity to feed your body the clean fuel it needs.

5 / Banish all processed goods.

Avoid anything that is chemically charged, overprocessed and loaded with artificial ingredients or preservatives. Plants are meant to be eaten whole so that the entire package of nutrients can benefit the human body.

6 / Drink three liters of water per day (at least!).

Water helps your body assimilate vitamins, minerals and macronutrients, it flushes out toxins and waste, and it increases your metabolism. It also keeps you full and less likely to reach for calorie-laden juices and sodas.

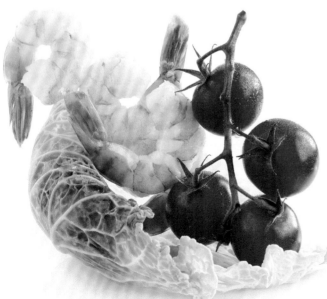

This power couple is your key to metabolism- and health-blasting results.

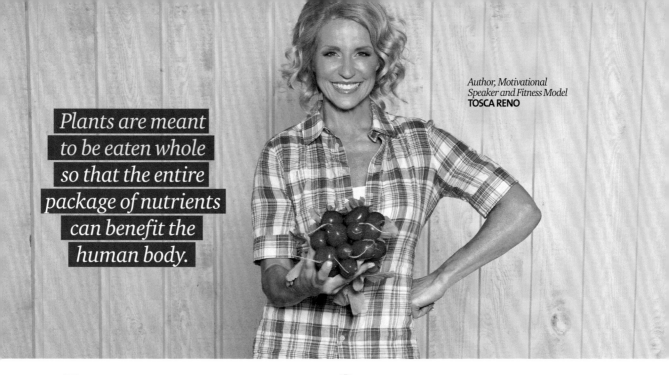

Plants are meant to be eaten whole so that the entire package of nutrients can benefit the human body.

Author, Motivational Speaker and Fitness Model
TOSCA RENO

7 / Portion size matters.

The beautiful thing about eating clean is that you're always carrying the perfect portion-measuring device with you – your hands. Here's how to get smart about food size:

ONE SERVING OF...	SHOULD FIT IN...
lean protein	the palm of your hand
leafy greens	two open hands cupped together
fruit and denser vegetables (e.g., beets & brussels sprouts)	one open hand
whole grains	one cupped hand

8 / Healthy fats are your friends.

Make sure you eat two or three servings of healthy fats per day. This can include nuts and seeds, along with coconut, olive, flaxseed and pumpkin seed oils to name a few. Healthy fats fill you up, stoke your metabolic rate, keep your hormones flowing and keep your brain functioning properly.

9 / Become a flexitarian.

Save money, reduce your carbon footprint and keep things interesting by choosing to prepare meatless meal options. Plant-based lean proteins include legumes, protein-dense grains such as quinoa, nuts, seeds, soy and seaweed.

10 / Carry a cooler.

Packing a day's worth of healthy eats is the best way to ensure that you will be sticking to your plan throughout the day. Timesaving tip: Choose one day of the week to prep your meals for the week and portion them out into small portable containers.

FIT TIP

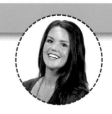

"I try and plan my meals as much as possible, and I bring food wherever I go. When I'm hungry and foodless I tend to make bad decisions!"

– Ashley Souter, designer

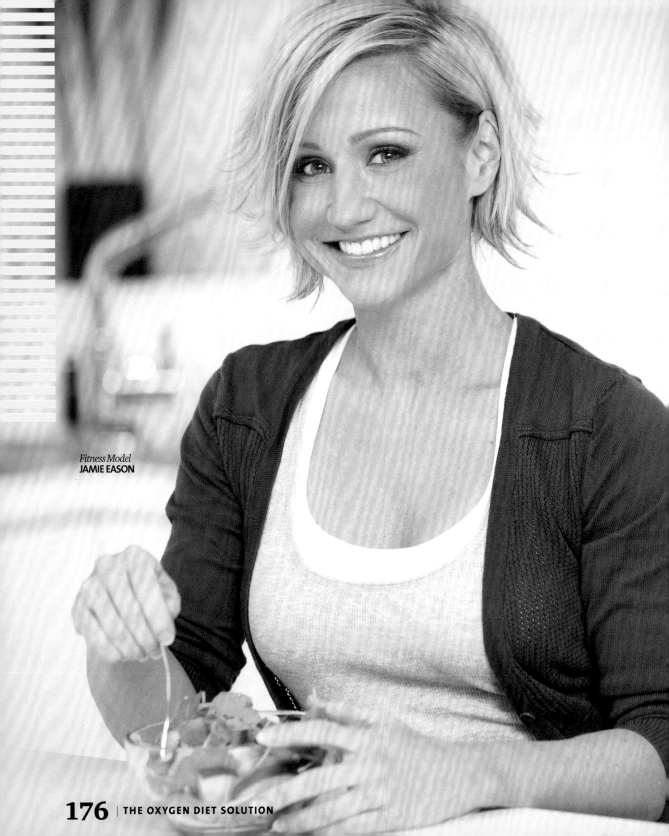

Fitness Model
JAMIE EASON

Calories Are Not Evil

JAMIE EASON SHOWS YOU HOW CALORIES ARE ON YOUR SIDE!

I have been known to be hardheaded at times. I can be so stubborn that if I swear a shirt I saw in a store was pink, and it is later presented before my eyes in what is clearly white, I would argue that it was off white, just to avoid defeat. Oh yeah, major hardhead! I like to think, however, that I have matured a lot over the years and have become far more pleasant and agreeable. Challenge that and you may regret it. OK, maybe I have a long way to go.

But I know I'm not the only headstrong one in my circle. I get it in return quite often, especially when I attempt to educate friends and family about living a fit lifestyle. Time and again, people claim to know what to do but then complain when it doesn't seem to be working. When I ask average women on the street what the basic principle is for losing weight I often hear, "Calories in versus calories out." They claim that they eat less and exercise more but never make any progress. Well, newsflash – that's the wrong approach! If that were in fact true, according to my caloric needs I could eat a few slices of carrot cake, my ultimate favorite dessert, and still be under my daily caloric requirement and not gain weight. I wish!

If we eat too many calories we will gain weight, but if we eat too few, we will likely end up experiencing the same fate. Drastically reducing calories can work for the short term but once our bodies catch on, they shift into preservation mode and the metabolism slows down to conserve energy. This perpetual dieting leads straight to a dead-end road. So, stop being so stubborn and eat!

The key is to retrain the brain to quit thinking of calories as "the bad guy." In most people's minds, calories equate to excess body fat. For years, I believed this to be gospel myself. However, according to *Webster's Medical Dictionary*, the definition of a calorie is "a unit representing the energy provided by food." Calories are energy, not evil demons lying in wait to pack on the pounds. When you think of it that way, it makes things way more clear.

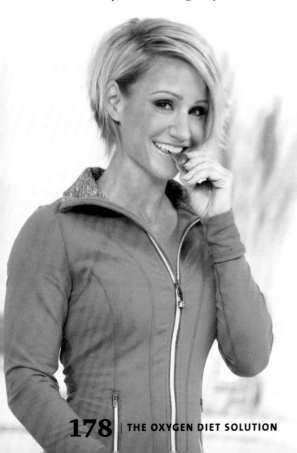

Most of us tend to be bargain shoppers. When we buy things, we typically set out to get the biggest bang for our buck, right? Then why not do this with our food? And I'm not talking about going to a buffet and stuffing yourself for $10.99, or to a restaurant where you can get bottomless bowls of pasta. We should be reading labels and studying the ingredients and making sure our grocery dollars are going toward the best items for our bodies. If you don't know the drill by now, this is the key – sticking with food that is unprocessed and unrefined is a far better way to consume your energy (and spend your hard-earned money).

> "*Eating the same all the time and denying my body the food it needs does nothing but set the stage for lethargy and misery.*"

Every person's caloric needs are highly individualized. We're all different and unless we know your specific weight and current training routine, it's hard to give an exact number. Someone training for a marathon or triathlon is going to require something completely different from someone aiming to lose the last 10 pounds or a figure model on the eve of a competition. Take me, for example. Sometimes I am like the Energizer Bunny and everything is go, go, go, and other times I get lucky enough to just take it easy and spend my day on the couch. Common sense would tell me on those high-energy days, I should be eating slightly more calories to accommodate the workload and slightly less on lower activity days. Yet, before I understood the need for sufficient fuel and the role it plays to keep my metabolism up and keep me lean, I admittedly would eat the same on both days. Eating the same all the time and denying my body the food it needs does nothing but set the stage for lethargy and misery.

There is a reason most fitness and nutrition experts recommend eating regular meals at even intervals throughout the day. *Oxygen*'s own nutrition expert and author of this book, Dr. Susan Kleiner, explains that when we eat regularly and our blood sugar stays on course, our bodies continue to build that precious muscle tissue, rather than tear it down.

"Metabolically, we run at a higher rate when we are anabolic, or in building mode, than when we are catabolic (tearing tissue down), which puts us in conservation mode," she says. She adds that when we're well fueled and our metabolisms are revving, our bodies are able to build muscle and burn more calories, which is what we want. "When we restrict calories too much, we become catabolic, which tears down muscle rather than build it, and lowers metabolic rate to conserve energy, burning fewer calories, even during exercise."

So, take some advice from this reformed hardhead and rethink your calories. The word "calorie" isn't a bad one. If you find that you are often tired or your progress has become stale, try increasing your calories rather than decreasing them. Eating the right foods more often is going to work. Plus, your mood and health – and of course your fitness – will all thank you for it!

JAMIE'S TIPS FOR FUELING UP

1. CHUG-A-LUG: Water and green tea are great to help squash hunger. Pair these with high-fiber foods and you'll keep hunger at bay longer.

2. KEEP SNACKS ON HAND: Be sure to plan ahead and bring healthy snacks wherever you go. This will keep you out of a situation where your only option is chips or a candy bar from the nearest vending machine.

3. EAT BREAKFAST: Get the metabolism revving bright and early. And don't say you don't have time. I hear this constantly. Get up 10 minutes earlier or get organized the night before. You definitely need your fuel to get your day going.

4. SLUMP BUSTERS: Wondering why you're not seeing results? Use a food journal to pinpoint where you might be straying from your meal plan.

5. DO YOUR HOMEWORK: Reading magazines like *Oxygen* and books like this one will get you on the right track and keep you there!

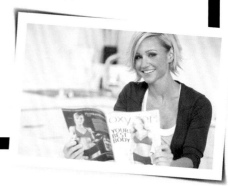

FIT TIP

"Simply flooding ourselves with poisonous foods disrespects the finely tuned nature of our cells."

– *Tosca Reno, author, motivational speaker and fitness model*

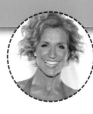

Diet Diagnosis

ARE THESE MISTAKES STOPPING YOU FROM MAXIMIZING MEALTIME RESULTS?

Working out regularly and eating right are part of every *Oxy* girl's game plan, of course, but if you're not seeing the results you want, it might be time for a tweak or two. Luckily we've compiled a day's worth of diet-related mistakes that will make it easy for you to identify where you might be going wrong. Once you discover the key ideas behind consuming the right foods at the right times throughout the day, you will be maximizing the way your body uses nutrients and responds to exercise – and, really, what could be better than that?

Breakfast Blunder:
Scrimping on the first meal of the day.

You've probably heard that filling your tank first thing in the morning is one of the most important things you can do, especially if you're looking to lose weight. While you sleep, your metabolism powers down and your body uses its stored energy in the form of glucose to repair itself and fuel your basic functions. When you wake up you need fuel to fire up that metabolism, energize your muscles and get your brain going – and a lonely bowl of cereal just isn't going to cut it. You need calories in the form of complex carbohydrates (to provide quick energy) and protein (to keep energy levels steady and help you stay full throughout the day). This will help you combat cravings and stave off bouts of impulsive, unplanned snacking, which can truly sabotage your weight-loss efforts.

In one study, researchers at Virginia Commonwealth University found that women who ate a healthy, protein-rich breakfast of up to 610 calories lost significantly more weight in eight months, and kept it off, compared to women who ate a scant 300-calorie breakfast. The meal plans in this book have been properly portioned out according to your goals, but as a rough breakfast guideline, try to aim for 10 to 15 grams of protein and at least 25 grams of carbohydrates (these numbers should be slightly higher if you are eating a preworkout breakfast).

When you wake up you need fuel to fire up that metabolism, energize your muscles and get your brain going.

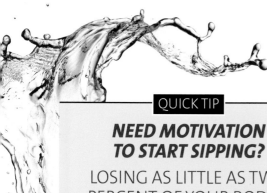

NEED MOTIVATION TO START SIPPING?

LOSING AS LITTLE AS TWO PERCENT OF YOUR BODY'S WATER VOLUME CAN LEAD TO MUSCLE WEAKNESS, FATIGUE AND IMPAIRED THINKING!

Preworkout Problem:
Running on empty.

Many people believe that working out on an empty stomach will help them burn fat, but this practice can actually do more harm than good. When you don't eat before exercising, especially first thing in the morning when your body has been fasting through the night, you put your system into a catabolic state. This means your body is forced to start breaking down your muscles because it doesn't have the resources to fuel them and build them back up.

To jumpstart the muscle-building process, you need to eat a small low-fat meal of roughly 15 to 20 grams of lean protein combined with 30 grams of carbohydrates about one hour before you work out. This will give your body enough time to start digesting, which will help you avoid cramps. Getting the amino acids found in protein into your system before you start breaking down muscle fibers during training ensures that protein is immediately and readily available to repair and rebuild the fibers.

If you don't have the time to eat an hour before working out, choose a small amount of something that is carb-based and easy to digest, such as a ripe banana with some yogurt or a smoothie with milk and berries (don't add the protein powder, though, as this is best for postworkout repair).

Training Dilemma:
Relying on store-bought energy drinks.

Getting your sweat on is a very good thing, but with all that perspiration and heavy breathing going on, you can lose a significant amount of water while working out. The trick to staying hydrated is to drink two cups of H_2O before your workout and continue sipping it throughout your sweat session.

Notice how we said water? Store-bought energy drinks often contain large amounts of sugar, which can lead to an insulin spike and subsequent crash. Instead of reaching for a sports drink, try adding a pinch of sea salt and a squeeze of lemon to your water. This super-hydrating cocktail will help your body replenish lost fluids and electrolytes without the sugar and chemical additives found in store-bought drinks.

NEED A TRICK TO HELP REDUCE THAT POSTWORKOUT PAIN?

TRY DRINKING 100% POMEGRANATE JUICE BEFORE HITTING THE GYM. RESEARCHERS AT THE UNIVERSITY OF TEXAS FOUND THAT WHEN PHYSICALLY FIT PEOPLE DRANK PURE POMEGRANATE JUICE FOR 15 DAYS AND THEN COMPLETED A STRENGTH-TRAINING WORKOUT, THEY HAD LESS POSTWORKOUT SORENESS AND WEAKNESS COMPARED TO THE PLACEBO GROUP. THE RESEARCHERS CLAIMED THE PHYTONUTRIENT ELLAGITANNIN WAS RESPONSIBLE FOR HELPING TO REDUCE INFLAMMATION.

After-Training Accident:
Missing the postworkout window of opportunity.

Just finished a stellar sweat session? Awesome! But now you've got to get some food in your system – stat! After working out, you have 30 to 60 minutes to take advantage of the one time when your muscles are depleted of fuel and will absorb anything you eat at an accelerated rate. This critical time period is called the "postworkout window of opportunity," and if you're looking to build lean muscle, avoid soreness and maintain ample energy stores, then you definitely don't want to miss it.

When refueling hungry muscles, consuming the right ratio of carbs to protein (roughly three parts carbs to one part protein) is essential. These carbs work in tandem with protein to support the muscle repair and rebuilding process, so always think of pairing your protein with an easily digested carbohydrate. You will also want to limit your intake of healthy fats at this meal, as it can slow down the absorption of nutrients. A fast and easy way to get this key carb/protein combo into your system is with a whey-based protein shake that contains fast-acting carbs (such as orange juice). This will fire up the recovery process and help replenish your body-fuel stores.

Dinnertime Don't:
Making it the main meal of the day.

If you want to lose weight, then you're going to have to rethink what is traditionally the heartiest meal of the day. And, when you think about it, getting the bulk of your calories early on in the day when you will have more opportunities to burn them off just makes sense. When you do eat your last meal of the day, a good rule of thumb is for 30 percent of your dinner calories to come from protein, 45 percent from carbs and the remainder from healthy fats. You should also eat your last meal three to four hours before bedtime. Speaking of shut-eye, make sure you get enough of it. A National Health and Nutrition Examination Survey involving 9,000 people revealed that individuals who averaged six hours of sleep per night were 27 percent more likely to be overweight than their counterparts who got seven to nine hours.

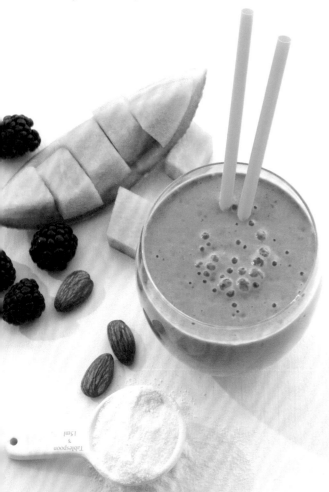

> *A fast and easy way of get this key carb/protein combo into your system is with a whey-based protein shake that contains fast-acting carbs.*

Nighttime No-No:
Succumbing to late-night cravings.

If you've followed all of this advice, namely the golden rule of combining complex carbs and lean protein at every meal, then your hunger levels should be quite manageable when the end of the day rolls around. However, even the best of us will sometimes have a hankering for a nighttime snack. The key is to keep it small – no more than 150 calories – and, again, make sure it consists of carbs and lean protein. The perfect nighttime nosh would be some low-fat Greek yogurt with berries. The high-quality carbs will raise mood-boosting serotonin levels, which will help you calm down before bed, and the slower-digesting protein from dairy will help your muscles kick into an anabolic, or muscle-building, state.

Dr. Susan's Tips on Treats

Although the meal plans allow for one treat per week and include Oxygen-approved suggestions, there may be occasions when you will want to enjoy one of your favorite foods instead. Don't worry! You can definitely plan to treat yourself without feeling like you've cheated (The concept of cheating doesn't fit with my philosophy – it's too negative and punitive!). You deserve it, after all, and your body will keep working just fine. Just make sure you stick to the following rules:

- **YOU CAN HAVE ONE** serving of a treat once per week – not a cheat day!
- **MAKE SURE YOU CHOOSE** something you absolutely love and savor it.
- **BE INFORMED** about what you are doing and make it a thoughtful choice.
- **A TREAT** that is a mix of carbs, fat and/or protein is better than a treat that is made up of only sugar/carbs (e.g., ice cream vs. hard candy).
- **NEED SUGGESTIONS?** Why not try a small square of dark chocolate (at least 70% cocoa) or a 5 oz glass of red wine? These both have health-boosting qualities – in moderation of course!

QUICK TIP

STILL HAVING TROUBLE DIAGNOSING YOUR DIET DILEMMAS?

TRY WRITING DOWN EVERYTHING YOU EAT IN A FOOD JOURNAL AND CROSS-REFERENCING IT WITH YOUR MEAL PLAN. YOU MIGHT BE SURPRISED BY WHAT YOU SEE!

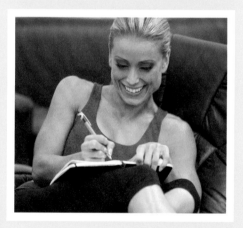

FIT TIP

"Knowing that my environment is stronger than my willpower, I always pre-plan my food far in advance. I save my 'treats' for when I'm out of the house. I do not allow any trigger foods past my front door or they don't stand a chance."

– *Lori Harder, fitness model*

Navigating the Grocery Store

We've probably all learned the hard way that shopping on an empty stomach is a major no-no (whether you're trying to save money or slim down), but did you know there is a whole cartload of simple shopping tips and tricks that should fill every *Oxy* gal's arsenal? For your shopping convenience, we've collected them in this handy guide. Read on, and in no time you'll be one savvy shopper!

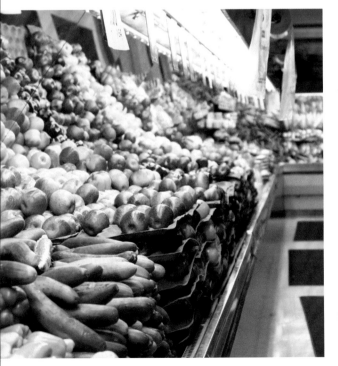

Don't forget your list!

A well-planned list that is organized to match the sections of the store will save you loads of time and money. And, if you promise yourself that you will stick to the list, you won't end up with a shopping cart full of expensive and unplanned junk food!

Use the wipes!

Most supermarkets offer sanitizing wipes near the store entrance – here's the reasoning: According to a 2011 University of Arizona study, 72 percent of the shopping carts tested had fecal matter on them and *E. coli* was discovered on 50 percent of the carts!

A well-planned list that is organized to match the sections of the store will save you loads of time and money.

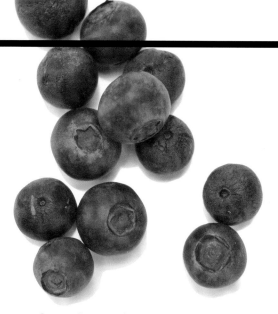

Shop the perimeter.

Have you ever noticed that the most nutritious foods – fresh veggies and fruits, dairy, lean meats, seafood and whole grains – are located around the edges of the store? If you make sticking to the perimeter one of your shopping strategies, you'll be less likely to suddenly find yourself in the candy aisle with a bag of M&M's in your hand.

Buy in season.

Just say no to expensive, imported fruits and veggies. Buying fresh, seasonal produce is cheaper, tastier and you'll be supporting local farmers and reducing your carbon footprint. If you're feeling like strawberries in the middle of winter, try frozen instead. You might even find a local variety, especially if you thought ahead in the summer and froze your own! They are just as nutritious and fresh – and they make great additions to smoothies!

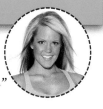

FIT TIP

"I try to eat foods that come from trees, the ground or an animal. If I can't pronounce the ingredients then it probably isn't the best choice."

– Nicole Wilkins, fitness model

GET TECHNICAL.

If you've got a smartphone or iPad, there are several apps to help with your strategic shopping and meal planning. Whether you need help with lists, coupons or price comparisons – there's an app for that. There's even an app called Food Essentials Scanner, which will scan an item's barcode to not only reveal information about calories, protein, and so on, but it can also be customized to instantly alert you to any allergens or ingredients you want to avoid.

"Using an app on my iPhone, I log all of my food intake when I am traveling for work or when I don't have home-cooked food in my travel bag – this takes the guesswork out of counting food nutritional values at pretty much any restaurant out there."

– Karen-Lisa Borders, fitness model

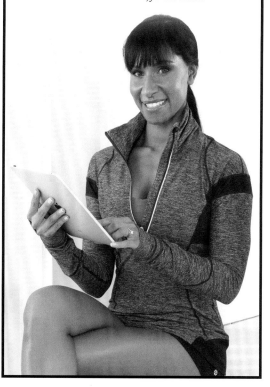

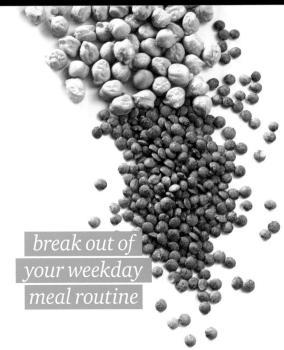

Make it meatless.

Choosing to make a vegetarian meal even one night a week will not only help you save money but is also the perfect way to break out of your weekday meal routine (or rut!). It's also great for your health – especially if you fill your cart with protein-packed meat alternatives like quinoa, legumes and eggs.

Make smart meat choices.

When you do buy meat, choose grass-fed, free-range meats that do not contain hormones and antibiotics. Meat from grass-fed animals has two to four times more heart-healthy omega-3s than meat from animals that are fed grains, and grass-fed is richer in antioxidants.

Read the labels.

Even if you've been diligent about shopping the perimeter, we know there will be times when you might have to detour into the inner aisles for some staples. So when you do, read the nutrition labels and ingredients carefully. Watch what actually constitutes a serving size (it is often smaller than you might think) and do your math accordingly. Ingredients to avoid: sugar (in all forms), partially hydrogenated oil, preservatives, chemicals and anything not found in nature.

break out of your weekday meal routine

Ingredients to avoid: sugar (in all forms), partially hydrogenated oil, preservatives, chemicals and anything not found in nature.

Don't fall for marketing tactics.

Once you're aware of them, you're less likely to fall victim to some of the tricky techniques marketers use to maximize profits. As soon as you set foot in the store you're inhaling the sweet aroma of freshly baked goods. Then there's the fact that staples like milk and eggs are at the back of the store. And as you make your way back there, you've got to resist all those tempting endcap displays, colorful packages and "huge" markdowns. You should also remember that the most expensive items are displayed at eye level. Look a little higher and lower and you will usually find cheaper options.

Check your receipts.

It sounds simple enough, but you can save a lot of money and hassle by checking your receipt before you leave the store. According to one study, 20 percent of consumers are overcharged at the checkout line – most often because some items are scanned more than once.

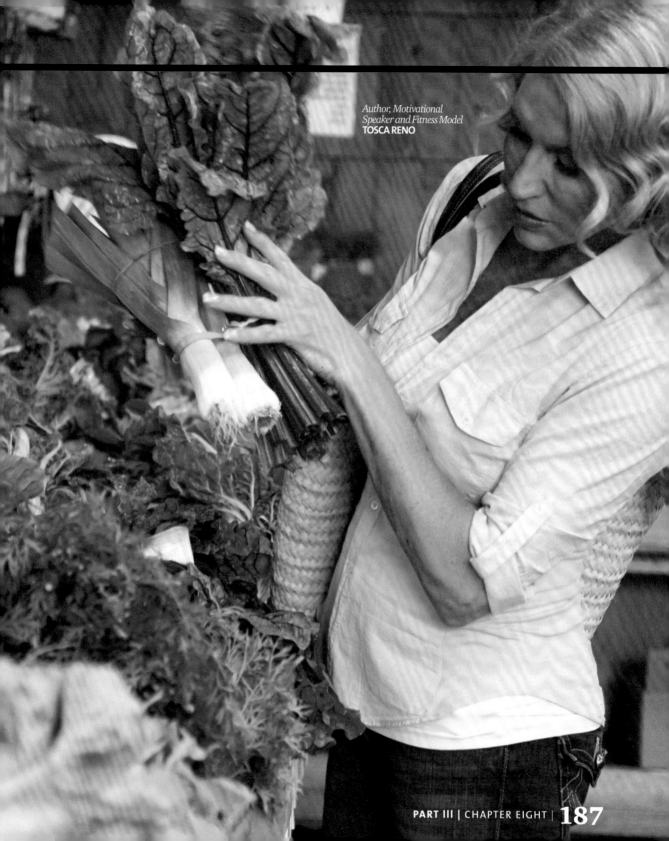

Author, Motivational
Speaker and Fitness Model
TOSCA RENO

The oxygen Diet Solution
Success Story

AFTER BUMPING HERSELF
UP ON HER PRIORITY LIST,
CINDY FLANNERY LOST
OVER 70 POUNDS!

"If I can do it, anybody can!"

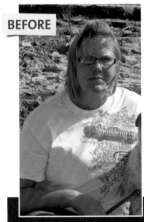

BEFORE

BEFORE: 230 lb
NOW: 156 lb
AGE: 38
HEIGHT: 5'5"
LOCATION: Austin, TX
OCCUPATION: Veterinary technician
FAVORITE EXERCISE: Biceps

A busy mom of three, Cindy Flannery always found the time to do it all – except fit in time for herself. She needed a change. "Without being healthy or physically fit, I'm nothing to my kids," she says. "It took me a long time to realize that."

Rude Awakening

When a stranger made a comment about her weight while shopping, Cindy transformed the negative experience into a positive push to finally change her ways, and would even consider thanking that same woman if she saw her again today! "I didn't want people to perceive me as being overweight or as teaching my children that it was OK," she says.

"I didn't want people to perceive me as being overweight or as teaching my children that it was OK."

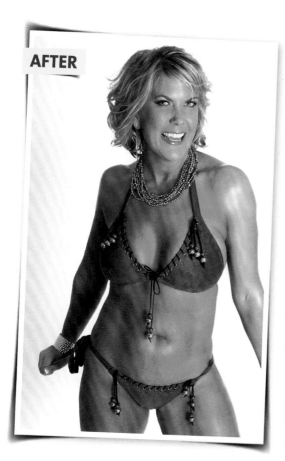

AFTER

Rise Before Dawn

Setting 4 a.m. dates with some sweat and iron at the gym, Cindy doesn't lack discipline. With an early bedtime, her meals and bag packed and ready to go by the door the night before, she's ready to take on the world when her alarm goes off. "My feet hit the ground running." With nobody standing in her way, Cindy finally feels great about herself.

Workout Time

Cindy switches up her cardio every day and alternates her lifting between heavy, low reps and lighter, high reps every six weeks. Here's how she stays on top when it comes to fitness:

MONDAY	Shoulders & cardio
TUESDAY	Plyo circuit & cardio
WEDNESDAY	Back, biceps & cardio
THURSDAY	Chest, triceps & cardio
FRIDAY	Rest
SATURDAY	Plyo circuit & cardio
SUNDAY	Legs

Support Team

Since day one, Cindy has had a team of people behind her while she put in hard hours at the gym and tossed junk food from her cupboards. She says she especially owes it to a few of her favorite guys for always rooting for her from the sidelines and even reminding her to have a protein shake from time to time. "My sons have been my biggest motivators, my biggest support staff, my cheerleaders, my coaches – they've been everything," she says of her children, aged seven, nine and 21.

Salad Makeover

Cindy loves Mexican food, but this modified taco salad is a fiesta without the guilt. "I could eat it for breakfast, lunch and dinner."

1. Brown extra lean ground turkey in a saucepan. Add a low-sodium taco seasoning to meat.

2. Serve over shredded lettuce with an ounce of avocado.

3. Add hot sauce (optional). "I put hot sauce on everything."

4. If desired, crumble a tortilla on top and enjoy.

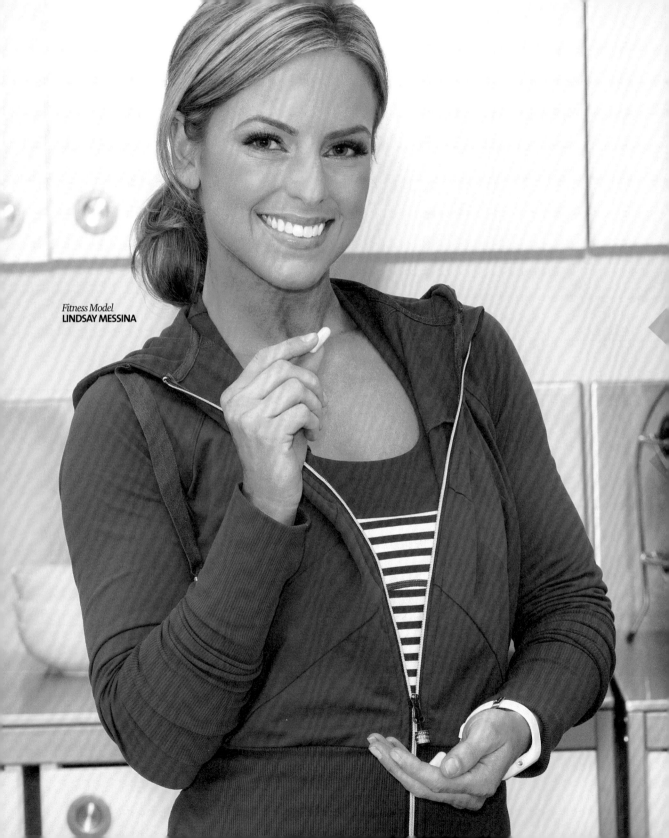

Fitness Model
LINDSAY MESSINA

Your Guide To Supplements

The best choices to power up your progress

Thermogenic amplifiers! Anti-catabolic BCAAs! Clinically proven! When it comes to the wide world of supplementation – and especially the claims made by some advertisements – it's enough to overwhelm and confuse anyone. If you've ever wondered about whether or not to include supplements in your diet or where they fit in the *Oxygen* lifestyle, you've come to the right place. This guide will help you make the best choice about what works for you. Just remember, supplements are the sidekicks to a regular diet and shouldn't be used to replace your daily requirements of macronutrients or micronutrients from food.

Creatine

WHAT: Creatine is a crystalline substance synthesized by amino acids and found in muscle tissue. It's known for reducing muscle damage and enhancing muscle growth, strength and power. As an antioxidant, it also aids in improving recovery and preserving lean muscles.

WHY TAKE IT: Creatine helps build and maintain lean muscle tissue, while also increasing muscle strength, power and mass. Creatine helps you train at a higher intensity and volume and offers a faster recovery time between sets. It also improves the anaerobic threshold (the maximum amount of high-intensity exercise you can do before your muscles run out of energy and begin to produce lactic acid). This delays the rate at which your muscles tire, meaning you can train harder, for longer.

DOSAGE: Consume three to five grams of creatine daily to load muscle stores.

WHERE TO GET IT: Creatine can be formed in your body after eating animal protein, including seafood (although you'd need to eat two pounds of meat to get three grams of creatine). Vegetarians can also make creatine, but in much smaller amounts. It can also be ingested as a supplement in powder, pill or liquid form. The best form is creatine monohydrate (the most natural form of creatine) with no added sugars or other ingredients. Powdered creatine is absorbed more quickly than in pill form. Creatine from vegan sources is also available.

SAFETY: Dosages exceeding five grams of creatine can produce side effects including gastrointestinal issues, muscle cramps, bad breath, strains, pains and dizziness. These side effects, even at 20 grams per day, are exceedingly rare. Creatine is increasingly being used to help people with various diseases such as Parkinson's and muscular dystrophy, and it is also used to help increase strength and endurance in those with heart disease.

Creatine helps us build and maintain lean muscle tissue, while also increasing muscle strength, power and mass.

Amino Acids

Amino acids are the building blocks of protein, which helps to build and repair muscles. Each amino acid is classified as either essential or non-essential. There are about 12 non-essential amino acids that are produced in your body and eight essential amino acids that you need to get from your diet. Glutamine is classified as a conditionally essential amino acid, which means your body produces limited amounts but you need to get extra in your diet in certain situations (such as after an intense workout or injury).

Branched-Chain Amino Acids (BCAAs)

WHAT: BCAAs contain leucine, isoleucine and valine, three of the eight essential amino acids. They are directly metabolized in your muscles, which means they have to pass through the liver. They act like a standby fuel (for muscle growth and recovery while you're resting) when they are sent directly to your muscle tissue.

WHY TAKE IT: If you do not have enough available BCAAs, your body will break down muscle tissue in order to get what it needs. These supplements help protect against muscle breakdown by reducing cortisol levels (the hormone that breaks down muscle tissue). They also promote muscle growth by kick-starting muscle synthesis (the creation of muscle tissue). BCAAs, particularly leucine, can also help burn through fat stores as a result of protein synthesis, which draws on fat stores to fuel muscle building. Leucine has been shown to decrease appetite, probably because having extra leucine convinces your brain that there is enough to do the job of muscle creation. These amino acids automatically increase the amount of energy the body has available during workouts. Valine actually increases energy by altering the way tryptophan behaves, by preventing it from signalling to the brain that the body is tired. It also increases muscle strength.

DOSAGE: Take three doses of three to five grams per day. Take one dose at breakfast, one 30 minutes before a workout and one within 30 minutes after a workout. They come in tablets, soft gels, capsules and powder form. These supplements are recommended for both before and after your workouts for muscle stamina and recovery.

WHERE TO GET IT: Chicken, eggs, fish, dairy products, beef and pork are animal sources. Vegetarian sources include legumes, nuts and seeds and whole grains.

SAFETY: Avoid use during pregnancy or when facing surgery (since glutamine impacts blood sugar). Check with a physician if you're taking diabetes medication. Don't take these supplements if using corticosteroids or thyroid medication.

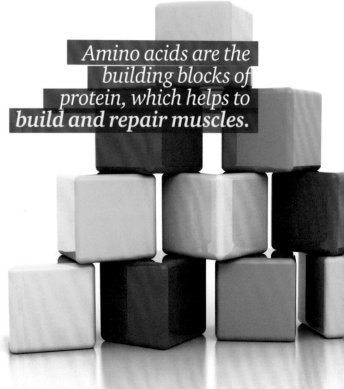

Amino acids are the building blocks of protein, which helps to build and repair muscles.

Conditionally Essential Amino Acid: Glutamine

WHAT: Glutamine is the most abundant non-essential amino acid, and is considered by experts to be a conditional non-essential amino acid. Normally our bodies produce enough, but in cases of acute recovery – after serious injuries, operations, severe burns or intense training – we may need to supplement. The primary fuel source for the immune system, glutamine is stored in the muscles. Depending on the intensity of your workout, exercise can deplete glutamine stores, promoting the breakdown of muscle tissue.

WHY TAKE IT: Glutamine helps optimize recovery in four ways. First, it prevents the body from using muscle tissue as fuel; this is known as protein sparing. It also stimulates the formation of glycogen (which your body gets from carbohydrates and uses as energy). Glutamine is important for cellular hydration, enhancing the process of building and repairing muscle tissue. Lastly, it protects the immune system since it's the top fuel source for immune cells, which help repair and build muscles. Glutamine can help you retain muscle mass and enhance recovery only if you're working out hard enough at your own fitness level. It is considered optimal for fitness competitors and endurance athletes.

DOSAGE: Take glutamine powder postworkout when your stores are likely depleted. Pills are large and expensive, while the powder is tasteless and blends easily with liquid. Mix three to six grams of glutamine with water or a quality whey protein and consume 30 to 60 minutes after training.

WHERE TO GET IT: Animal products, including meat, fish and dairy.

SAFETY: Glutamine may not be needed for active people who refuel with adequate amounts of carbs and protein. Exceeding 20 grams of glutamine per day could lead to gastrointestinal issues such as diarrhea. Do not mix with hot drinks because heat destroys glutamine. People with kidney or liver disease or undergoing cancer therapy should not take it. Consult a physician before consuming glutamine if taking medications.

The primary fuel source for the immune system, glutamine is stored in the muscles.

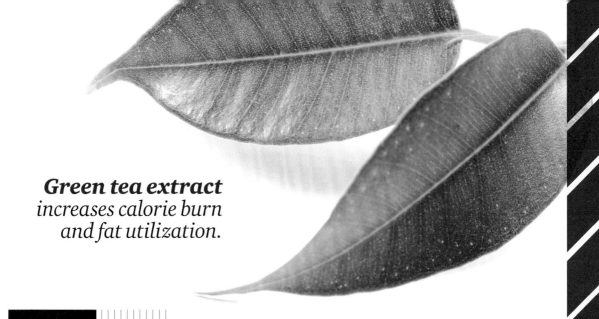

Green tea extract increases calorie burn and fat utilization.

Fat Burners

Fat burners are supplements that focus on increasing the body's metabolism in order to do just as you might imagine – help you burn fat. These supplements will increase the rate of your body's fat-burning potential without your having to increase your efforts.

Capsinoids

WHAT: Capsaicin is the compound that makes chile peppers spicy. Capsinoids are a relative of capsaicin but without the burn.

WHY TAKE IT: Capsinoids boost your body's ability to burn more calories and have been shown to suppress appetite and burn belly fat. There are also potential benefits for total cholesterol and triglyceride levels.

DOSAGE: Six milligrams per day for 12 weeks.

WHERE DO YOU GET IT: Capsinoids are from sweet peppers, but you would have to eat an unrealistic amount to get the benefits. Supplements are ideal for getting the proper amount.

SAFETY: There are no safety concerns with capsinoids.

Green Tea Extract

WHAT: Caffeine and catechin epigallocatechin gallate (EGCG).

WHY TAKE IT: Green tea extract increases calorie burn and fat utilization. It may also cut the risk of developing heart disease because of its high levels of antioxidants.

DOSAGE: 270 milligrams EGCG + 150 milligrams caffeine per day, split into three doses before meals. Or drink up to five cups of green tea per day.

WHERE TO GET IT: Green tea and green tea extracts.

FIT TIP

"I take my essential fatty acids loyally to ensure everything – from fat loss to energy levels to nails and hair – is optimized!"

– Karen-Lisa Borders, fitness model

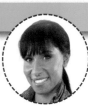

Conjugated Linoleic Acid (CLA)

WHAT: CLA is a family of fatty acids naturally found in beef and dairy foods. Supplements are made from safflower or sunflower oils, which contain a mixture of CLA-like chemical structures called isomers 9, 11 and 10, 12. Isomers 10, 12 have the greatest anti-obesity effect.

WHY TAKE IT: CLA diminishes the number of fat cells in the body. Animal studies have found benefits in bodyweight regulation, fat loss and lean-tissue maintenance. It may also increase bone mineral density.

DOSAGE: Four to six grams per day for three to six months.

WHERE TO GET IT: While CLA occurs naturally in grass-fed beef and dairy, you would have to eat such an extraordinary amount of these foods to get enough of this fatty acid that doing so would be impossible. Taking supplements is recommended.

SAFETY: When first taking CLA, some people experience nausea, gastrointestinal issues and diarrhea. However, these side effects can be reduced by taking the supplement with milk. Side effects will fade within the first two weeks of regular consumption. CLA may decrease HDL (good) cholesterol and insulin sensitivity. Do not take if diabetic or breastfeeding.

Fish Oil Capsules

WHAT: Fish oil capsules are made from oily fish that are high in omega-3 fatty acids, such as salmon, sardines and mackerel. If you dislike fish and seafood, taking fish oil supplements is an alternative way to get your dose of healthy fats. These supplements contain DHA (docosahexaenoic acid) and EPA (eicosapentaenoic acid), omega-3 fats that are key structural components in brain cells and are critically involved in anti-inflammatory functions in brain and body cells. When DHA is low, the brain slows down the loss of all fats in order to raise its availability in the body.

WHY TAKE IT: Studies have found that stomach fat decreases when subjects consume ample amounts of fish oil. Taking fish oil capsules will lower levels of cortisol, the fat-loving stress hormone, and will elevate your mood. These omega-3 fats are also a potent anti-inflammatory.

DOSAGE: About 500 to 1,000 milligrams of a combination of DHA and EPA per day. When buying fish oil capsules, make sure you read the label and take the recommended dosage.

WHERE TO GET IT: Fish oil can be taken in capsule form. Algal oil supplements contain a high level of DHA but each capsule contains a much smaller dose than fish oil capsules.

SAFETY: Fish oil supplements may occasionally cause a fishy aftertaste, fishy smelling burps and diarrhea (with very high doses). Do not take if you suffer from hemophilia, if you take blood thinning medication or if you are going to have surgery.

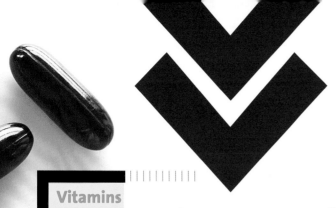
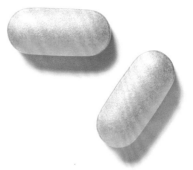

Vitamins

Getting a full spectrum of vitamins in your diet may be difficult if you rely on your nutrition plan alone. Taking vitamin supplements can help make up for micronutrients that are lacking in your diet. They are essential for anything from boosting your body's immunity to fighting off the signs of aging. Here are two you might consider taking.

Vitamin E

WHAT: Vitamin E is a powerful free-radical fighter that comes from healthful fatty foods. It occurs naturally as eight different chemicals in food.

WHY TAKE IT: Vitamin E plays a crucial role as an antioxidant in the human body. It works to slow the damage to our hearts, brains and eyes that naturally occurs with age. Vitamin E helps to keep your immune system healthy and acts as a natural anti-inflammatory, with benefits for everything from your arteries to your joints.

DOSAGE: A well-balanced diet that contains your daily dose of healthy fats, fruits and vegetables. One spoonful of wheat germ provides the recommended daily quota of 22 IU. Vitamin E is a fat-soluble vitamin, so make sure to consume fats when you take it.

WHERE TO GET IT: You can consume it naturally in healthy fatty food sources such as nuts, seeds and olive oil. You can also find it in fruits and vegetables such as broccoli, red peppers, kiwifruit, collard greens, mangoes and tomatoes.

SAFETY: Research shows it's best to obtain vitamin E from food sources because it is better tolerated.

Vitamin D

WHAT: Vitamin D is known as the sunshine vitamin, since our bodies produce it after exposure to sunshine. Vitamin D3 is needed to produce serotonin, the "feel-good" neurotransmitter in our brains. Most people who live above the latitude of Atlanta, Georgia, need a vitamin D3 supplement to help maintain a sense of wellbeing and energy throughout the winter.

WHY TAKE IT: The sun's UV rays stimulate a biochemical reaction on the skin to create vitamin D. Our vitamin D levels drop during the winter because of our reduced exposure to sunlight. This can dampen our mood. Vitamin D also improves bone health, muscle recovery and growth. Foods rich in vitamin D can help, but our absorption from food sources is fairly low.

DOSAGE: 1,000 to 2,000 IU of vitamin D3 daily during the winter.

WHERE TO GET IT: The sun, fish oil, salmon, mackerel, orange juice, fortified dairy products, beef liver, sardines, eggs, fortified cereal, squid, rainbow trout, bluefin tuna. It can also be taken as a supplement in pill form.

SAFETY: Taking large amounts of vitamin D supplements could result in hypocalcaemia (an excess of calcium in the blood). Symptoms include constipation, painful calcium deposits, loss of appetite, weakness and confusion. Avoid taking large doses if pregnant.

Protein Powder

Sometimes it's just not possible to cook a filet of fish or grill a chicken breast. This is where protein powders are a blessing. They are convenient and provide the dose of protein you need at any meal.

Whey

WHAT: Whey protein powder comes from milk and is a fast-digesting complete protein. It contains amino acids for muscle growth and recovery, including high amounts of branched-chain amino acids.

WHY TAKE IT: BCAAs are needed for muscle tissue maintenance and become depleted after exercise. Consuming whey right after a workout will help repair muscles, while also aiding in your body's production of disease-fighting antioxidants. It also helps to burn fat.

DOSAGE: One scoop, which usually contains about 25 to 30 grams of protein.

WHERE TO GET IT: Whey concentrates and whey isolates. Whey concentrates contain lactose (carbs) and fat from milk, while isolates contain only whey protein (ideal for those who are lactose intolerant).

SAFETY: Do not consume if you have an allergy or sensitivity to dairy. Twenty-five grams gives you an ideal amount to boost protein synthesis. Just make sure you rely on whole foods for the rest of your day's protein. Some people may experience gas and bloating from animal-based protein powders.

Casein

WHAT: Casein is a complete milk protein that prolongs the release of amino acids, helping to keep you feeling full between meals.

WHY TAKE IT: Casein reduces muscle damage that can occur 48 hours after a workout. It is also good to consume before bed, since the slow absorption supplies your body with protein through the night when it enters a catabolic state (breaks down protein for energy). Casein may boost immunity while helping to burn fat stores, because of its high amounts of glutamine.

DOSAGE: One scoop, which usually contains about 15 to 20 grams of protein.

WHERE TO GET IT: Buy micellar casein, a non-hydrolyzed form that retains the slow-release effect.

SAFETY: Do not consume if you are lactose intolerant. Your body doesn't need more than 25 grams of protein per meal, so there is no reason to go overboard with your serving size. Some people may experience gas and bloating from animal-based protein powders.

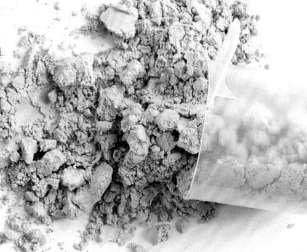

One scoop usually contains about 25 grams of protein

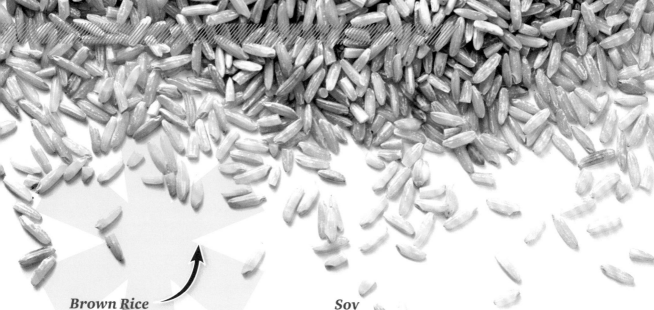

Brown Rice

WHAT: As a plant protein, brown rice is incomplete because it lacks one essential amino acid, lysine, which helps manage triglycerides (a form of body fat), and is needed for hormone production and bone growth.

WHY TAKE IT: Brown rice protein powder can be used by vegans and vegetarians, or for anyone trying to cut down on their consumption of animal products. To make up for the lack of lysine, you can pair brown rice protein powder with milk or soy. Brown rice protein powder absorbs readily, and is easily tolerated by people who are lactose intolerant or have a sensitive stomach.

DOSAGE: One scoop, which usually contains about 15 grams of protein. It must be taken with milk or soy to make it a complete protein.

WHERE TO GET IT: Brown rice protein powder.

SAFETY: Your body will need the additional protein source pairing for lysine to fully utilize the rice protein.

Soy

WHAT: This vegetarian protein source comes from soybeans and is best for women.

WHY TAKE IT: Soy compounds known as isoflavones can combat menopausal symptoms and reduce the risk of breast cancer. It also aids in fat burning.

DOSAGE: One scoop, which usually contains about 20 to 25 grams of protein.

WHERE TO GET IT: Soy isolates contain more isoflavones and less fat and cholesterol than soy concentrates.

SAFETY: Soy should not be eaten in large amounts because it contains plant compounds called isoflavones, which mimic the sex hormone estrogen. Consuming too much soy may lead to reduced fertility in women and affect the development of fetuses in pregnant women. A high soy intake may also decrease testosterone levels in men. People with thyroid disorders should avoid large doses of soy products. Absorption of nutrients such as zinc, iron and calcium may be reduced. Consuming soy products may not be safe for women who have suffered from breast cancer, are pregnant or taking oral contraceptives. It's best to speak with a physician before taking soy protein, and to use in moderation.

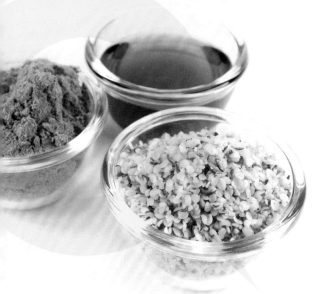

Hemp

WHAT: A great protein source for vegans, hemp protein powder comes from whole hempseeds, which contain about 25 percent highly digestible protein.

WHY TAKE IT: Hemp protein powder offers a good dose of the anti-inflammatory group of essential fatty acids, omega-3s, which aid in muscle recovery after a workout. However, hemp protein powder is not considered a complete protein. Simply adding a variety of plant proteins to your diet throughout the day can make up for this. Hemp helps your heart by lowering cholesterol levels with its fiber content, and its omega-3s enhance memory, focus and concentration.

DOSAGE: One scoop, which contains about 10 grams of protein. Pair hemp with beans, legumes and grains to provide all the essential amino acids needed to complete the protein.

WHERE TO GET IT: Hempseeds.

SAFETY: You must have other sources of protein to create complete proteins for your body to use daily. The omega-3 fats in hemp are excellent anti-inflammatory compounds, but do not substitute for DHA and EPA found in fish oil.

Natural Supplements

Supplements don't always come in pill or powder form. Nature offers her own tidbits of vitamins, minerals, healthy fats and more in something as small as a flaxseed. Power up your diet with these natural wonders.

Flaxseed

WHAT: Flaxseed is a plant seed high in omega-3 fatty acids such as alpha-linolenic acid (ALA), which the body cannot produce.

WHY TAKE IT: Flaxseed can lower the risk of certain types of cancer. It can also aid in the regulation of blood sugar and help lower cholesterol and blood pressure. Flaxseed also increases your metabolic rate and helps keep you regular. For women, flaxseed has been reported to help with menopausal symptoms, enhance the immune system and alleviate inflammatory conditions.

DOSAGE: One to two tablespoons of ground flaxseed per day.

WHERE TO GET IT: Buy flaxseeds whole and grind them before you consume. If you don't, the seeds will pass through your intestine without the nutrients being absorbed. Store them in the fridge.

SAFETY: Start with one tablespoon per day of ground flaxseed and work your way up to two tablespoons per day. Flaxseed can cause gastrointestinal issues such as diarrhea if taken in excess.

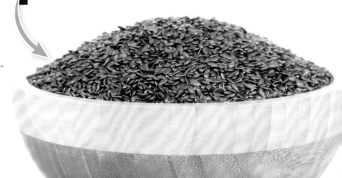

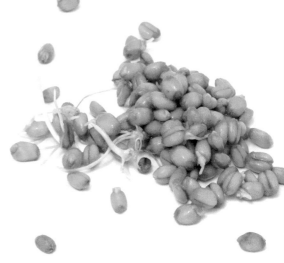

Wheat Germ

WHAT: Wheat germ is the part of the wheat kernel that germinates. It is the most nutrient-dense part of the kernel, and contains the majority of its fat.

WHY TAKE IT: Wheat germ is a nutritional power-house with a high amount of B vitamins, vitamin E, omega-3 fatty acids, minerals and fiber. Studies have shown it protects against cardiovascular disease, regulates blood sugar, is high in antioxidants and helps to regulate blood pressure and bowel function.

DOSAGE: Two tablespoons per day.

WHERE TO GET IT: Wheat germ and whole wheat products.

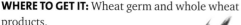

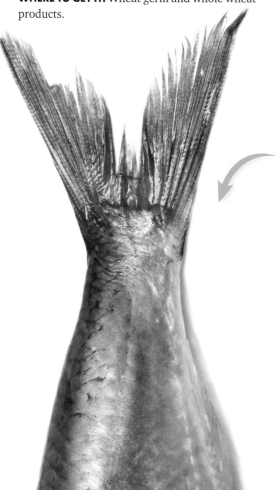

Fatty Fish

WHAT: Fatty fish, such as salmon, contain healthy fats that your brain needs to function properly. They are chock full of two kinds of omega-3 fatty acids: DHA (docosahexaenoic acid) and EPA (eicosapentaenoic acid). These fats are powerful anti-inflammatory agents.

WHY TAKE IT: Fatty fish contain DHA, which helps to keep the brain cell membrane pliable and reduces inflammation that could cause damage. This is essential for the maintenance of memory, cognitive function, mental focus and mental energy. The healthy fats from fish have also been proven to combat belly fat. Low levels of DHA and EPA are linked to the development of depression and post-partum depression. So overall, eating fatty fish each week will boost your mood!

DOSAGE: Eat five ounces of fatty fish three to five times per week.

WHERE TO GET IT: Any cold water fatty fish. Salmon, herring, mackerel, halibut, lake trout, sardines, tuna and whitefish are the best sources.

SAFETY: Fish may contain mercury. Depending on the specific fish eaten, pregnant women and those nursing may need to limit their consumption to one meal of fish per week. Wild-caught Pacific salmon is an excellent choice.

The Inside Scoop

OXYGEN EDITORS SHARE THEIR SUPPLEMENTATION SECRETS!

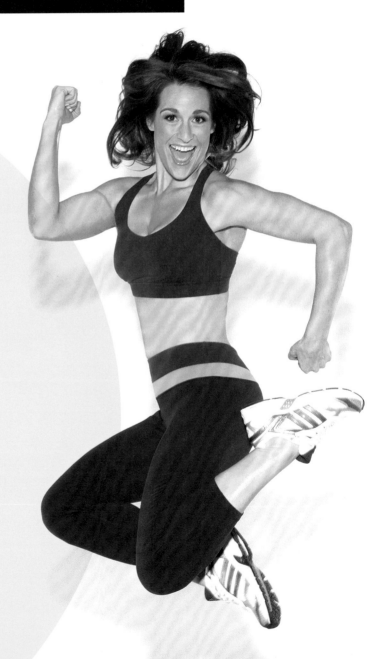

"I used to think my daily multivitamin was all the supplement I needed. When I joined the Oxygen team and started training for muscle building and fat loss, I learned there was a whole world of pills and powders that could help me hit those goals. Now I use whey powder daily for a quick hit of protein and a long list of amino acids. BCAAs are essential preworkout for muscle maintenance and endurance, glutamine postworkout for quicker recovery, and when I have a really hard workout planned, a little creatine for energy and muscle building goes a long way. But the one supplement I can't imagine giving up? Those omega-3 packed super-pills: high-quality fish oil!"

— KIRSTYN BROWN, NUTRITION EDITOR

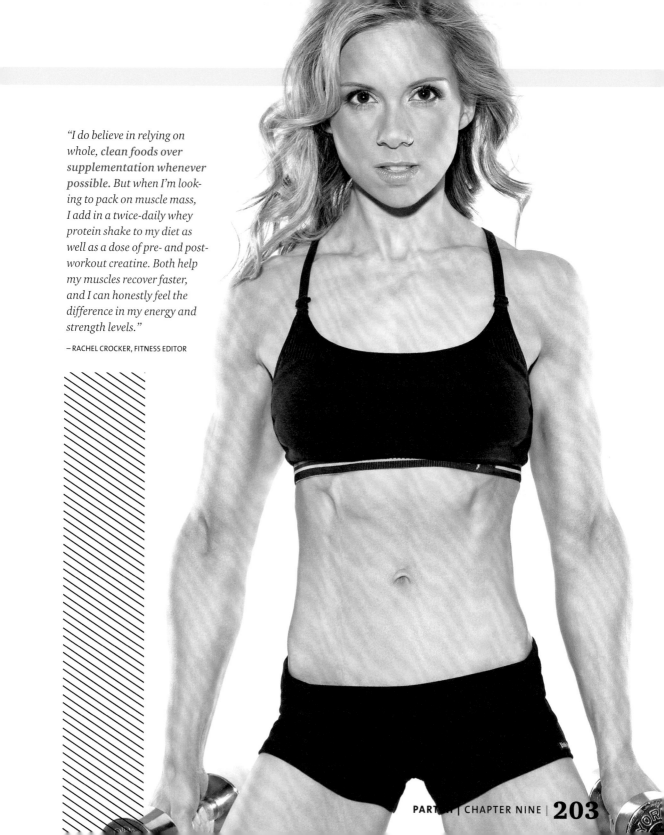

"I do believe in relying on whole, clean foods over supplementation whenever possible. But when I'm looking to pack on muscle mass, I add in a twice-daily whey protein shake to my diet as well as a dose of pre- and post-workout creatine. Both help my muscles recover faster, and I can honestly feel the difference in my energy and strength levels."

– RACHEL CROCKER, FITNESS EDITOR

The oxygen Diet Solution Success Story

WITH VISIONS OF MUSCLES AND PHYSICAL FEATS, MYLENE BIDDLE TOOK ON THE WEIGHT ROOM AND DROPPED 35 POUNDS.

"I am a strong woman!"

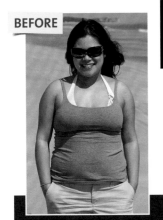

BEFORE

BEFORE: 165 lb
NOW: 130 lb
AGE: 27
HEIGHT: 5'2"
LOCATION: Crestview, FL
OCCUPATION: Software engineer
FAVORITE EXERCISE: Wide-legged squat on the rack

When Mylene Biddle struggles while lifting at the gym, she turns to visualization. "I think of pro bodybuilder Ronnie Coleman's saying, 'Ain't nothing but a peanut!' and envision the weight as a tiny peanut," she laughs. "Then I lift it." These days, there isn't much Mylene can't do. Over the past two years, she's dropped 35 pounds and, last year, strutted her stuff on stage at an NPC bikini competition.

Muscles on her mind

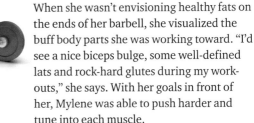

When she wasn't envisioning healthy fats on the ends of her barbell, she visualized the buff body parts she was working toward. "I'd see a nice biceps bulge, some well-defined lats and rock-hard glutes during my workouts," she says. With her goals in front of her, Mylene was able to push harder and tune into each muscle.

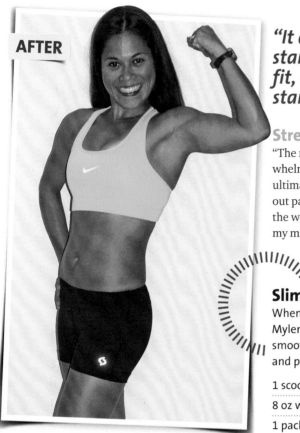

AFTER

"It doesn't matter how you start on becoming healthy and fit, as long as you start, and start now. Seize the day!" "

Stress buster

"The more stressed out I am, the more I feel overwhelmed with my fitness goals," says Mylene. Her ultimate way to overcome stress and stay fit? A workout partner with a wagging tail. "A nice hike through the woods with my dog, Buster, really helps to clear my mind and balance my emotions," she says.

Slimming Sip

When she craves something sweet in the evenings, Mylene turns to her version of a frappuccino smoothie. She blends up the following ingredients, and puts a cap on that sweet tooth:

1 scoop vanilla protein powder

8 oz water or almond milk

1 packet of decaf instant coffee

Ice

Stevia, to taste

TRY ADDING NATURAL PEANUT BUTTER!

Pulling it off

"I really didn't think I'd ever be able to do pull-ups," says Mylene. "The day I grabbed the bar and knocked out three of them in a row, I was so overwhelmed that I stood there, staring at the bar in disbelief for a couple of minutes!" With a newfound sense of pride and boosted confidence, Mylene knew at that moment that she was converted from a cardio queen to a Sister in Iron.

Seeing herself fit

Looking ahead to the future, Mylene sees an even fitter self. With a new love for CrossFit, she's finding fresh ways to challenge both her muscles and her imagination. If she can envision it, she says, it ain't nothing but a peanut.

Move Like Mylene

Mylene trains six days a week, beginning every workout with cardio. She then splits her strength training into the following routines:

MONDAY: Legs
TUESDAY: Shoulders
WEDNESDAY: Back & Biceps
THURSDAY: Glutes & Legs
FRIDAY: Chest, Abs & Triceps
SATURDAY: Shoulders & Calves
SUNDAY: Rest

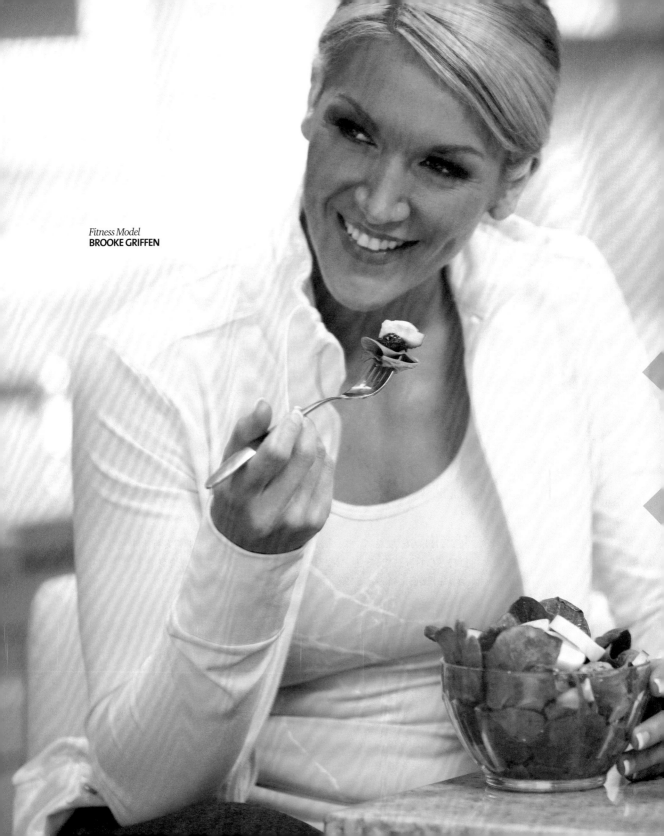

Recipes

If this section of the book had a slogan, it could be something along the lines of "Come for the science, stay for the flavor."

In other words, the science of nutrient timing and combining is what makes these meals effective, but it's the emphasis on mouthwateringly fresh ingredients with minimal prep work that makes them irresistible. So, although you will become familiar with these recipes as you follow the meal plans, we're sure they'll earn a permanent spot in your repertoire – especially since most of them are ready in 30 minutes or less!

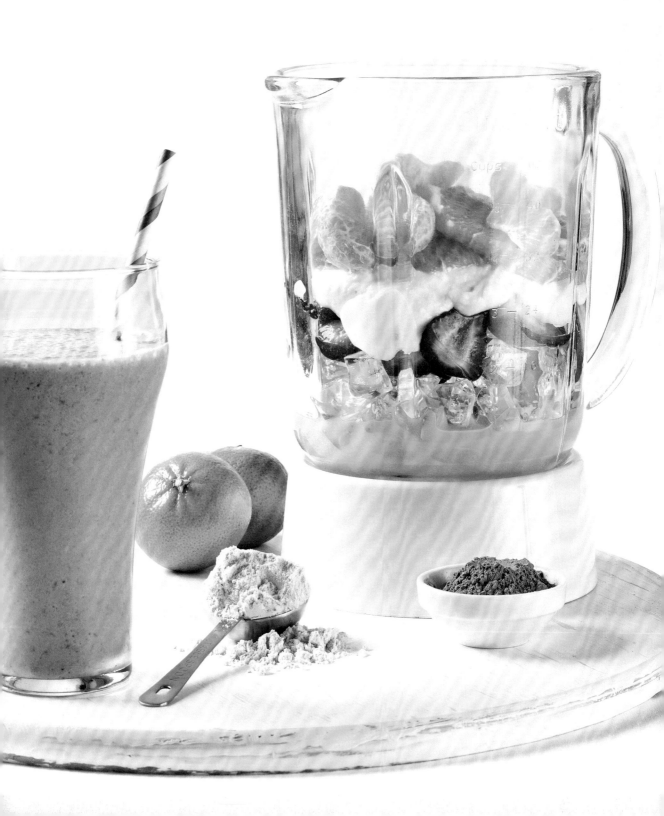

SUNSHINE
BREAKFAST SHAKE

Ready in 5 minutes
Makes 2 servings

½ peeled navel orange
2 peeled mandarin oranges
½ cup frozen strawberries
7 oz 100% orange juice
1 tsp matcha green tea
1 scoop whey protein isolate powder
½ cup plain low-fat yogurt
Ice cubes

Blend all ingredients in a blender.

FIT FACT: *Combining citrus with green tea helps the body better absorb more of the tea's beneficial flavonoids.*

Nutrients per serving:

Calories: 200, Total Fats: 2 g,

Saturated Fat: 1 g, Trans Fat: 0 g,

Cholesterol: 20 mg, Sodium: 65 mg,

Total Carbohydrates: 34 g,

Dietary Fiber: 3 g, Sugars: 26 g,

Protein: 14 g, Iron: 1 mg

BANANA-WALNUT PROTEIN PANCAKES

Ready in 20 minutes
Makes 8 pancakes

3 small bananas, very ripe
½ cup chopped walnuts
6 egg whites

DRY INGREDIENTS:
1 cup rolled oats
1 tbsp ground flaxseed
1 tbsp wheat germ
2 tbsp protein powder
2 tsp ground cinnamon
½ tsp sea salt

WET INGREDIENTS:
1 tsp vanilla
2 tsp maple syrup
½ cup plain low-fat Greek yogurt

1. In a large bowl, mash bananas until smooth. Add walnuts; set aside.

2. In a separate bowl, beat egg whites until stiff. Set aside.

3. In a large prep bowl, combine dry ingredients.

4. Add wet ingredients to the bananas. Mix well. Fold in egg whites. Add the dry ingredients to wet and mix gently to combine.

5. Heat a skillet on medium-high heat with a light coating of cooking oil (canola or coconut). Pour about ¼ cup of batter for each pancake. Cook on one side until bubbles appear on top, then flip to cook the other side, about 2 minutes per side. Repeat until all batter has been used up. Serve.

Nutrients per pancake:

Calories: 160, Total Fats: 6 g,

Saturated Fat: 1 g, Trans Fat: 0 g,

Cholesterol: 0 mg, Sodium: 180 mg,

Total Carbohydrates: 20 g,

Dietary Fiber: 3 g, Sugars: 6 g,

Protein: 9 g, Iron: 3 mg

FIT FACT: *Bananas contain resistant starch, which studies suggest nudges your body to use up fat for energy instead of carbs.*

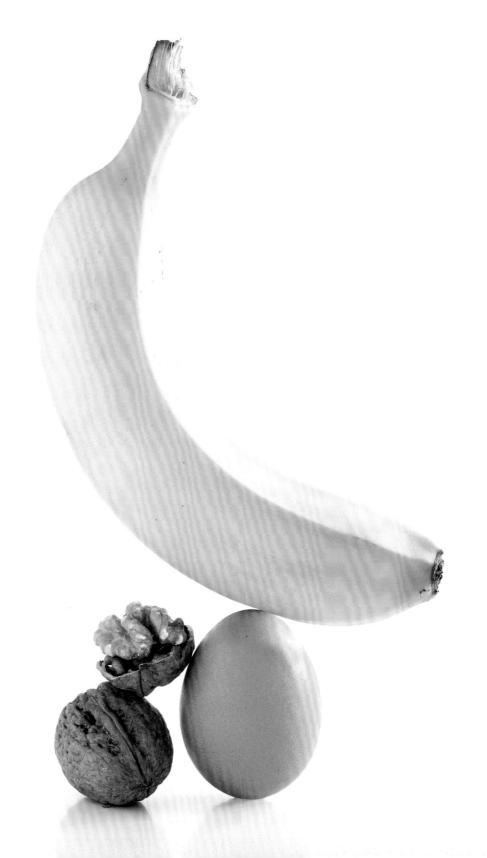

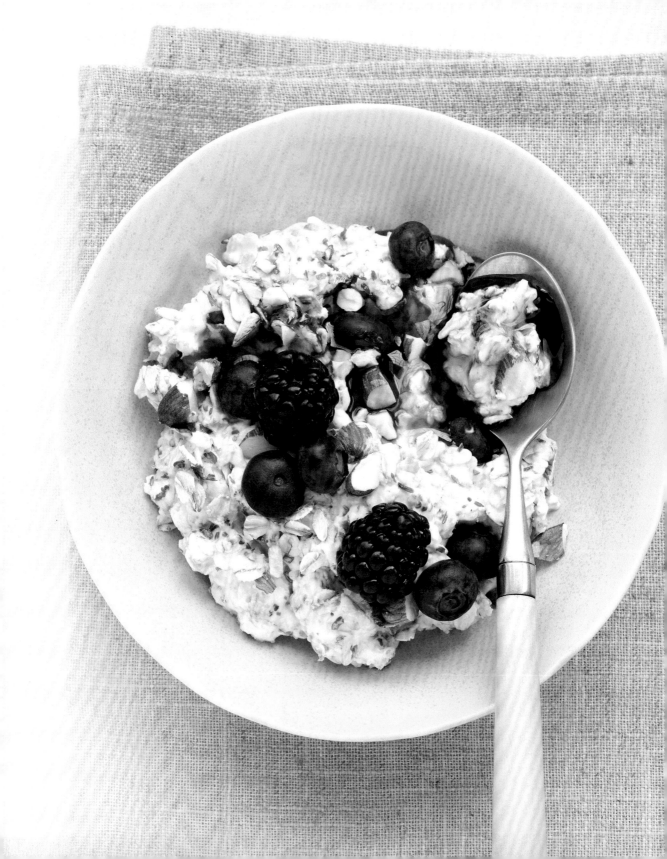

IMMUNITY-BOOSTING MUESLI

*Ready in 5 minutes (not
including overnight prep)
Makes 2 servings*

½ cup old-fashioned oats
1 cup plain nonfat Greek yogurt
1 tbsp ground flaxseeds
1 tbsp crushed almonds
1 tsp cinnamon
1 tbsp 100% maple syrup
1 cup fresh mixed berries

1. Stir oats into yogurt.

2. Mix in ground flaxseeds and crushed almonds.

3. Stir in cinnamon and mix.

4. Stir in syrup and add berries. Refrigerate overnight.

FIT FACT: *Ground flaxseeds are the richest plant source of the
inflammation-fighting omega-3 fatty acids. They contain fiber,
which improves insulin sensitivity and wards off fat build-up.*

Nutrients per serving:

Calories: 242, Total Fats: 5 g,

Saturated Fat: 0.5 g, Trans Fat: 0 g,

Cholesterol: 0 g, Sodium: 36 mg,

Total Carbohydrates: 36 g,

Dietary Fiber: 5 g, Sugars: 18 g,

Protein: 16 g, Iron: 1 mg

APPLE-OATMEAL CHOCOLATE PROTEIN BARS

Ready in 40 minutes
Makes 6 servings

2 cups rolled oats
½ cup natural nut butter
1 tbsp coconut oil
1 tbsp ground flaxseed
4 scoops chocolate protein powder
½ cup unsweetened applesauce
   (add more if mix is too dry)

1. Line an 8-inch square baking dish with parchment paper.

2. Combine all ingredients in a medium-sized mixing bowl. Use clean hands to mix the ingredients until they are well blended.

3. Pour mixture into lined dish and smooth with the back of a spoon until even.

4. Place in freezer for 30 minutes. Remove from freezer and cut into 6 bars. Serve.

FIT TIP: *Protein powder is a convenient source of amino acids, the building blocks of muscle. Best for baking: whey or soy.*

FIT FACT: *Apples provide waist-whittling pectin fiber, and using applesauce as a substitute for vegetable oils when baking cuts down on fat content dramatically.*

Nutrients per serving:
Calories: 330, Total Fats: 16 g,
Saturated Fat: 4 g, Trans Fat: 0 g,
Cholesterol: 30 mg, Sodium: 45 mg,
Total Carbohydrates: 28 g,
Dietary Fiber: 6 g, Sugars: 5 g,
Protein: 22 g, Iron: 1.5 mg

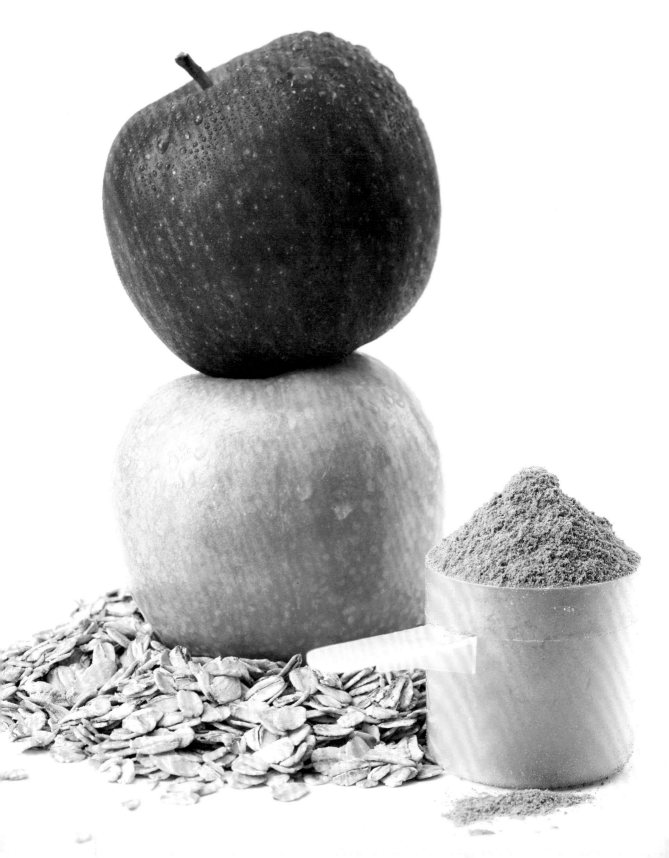

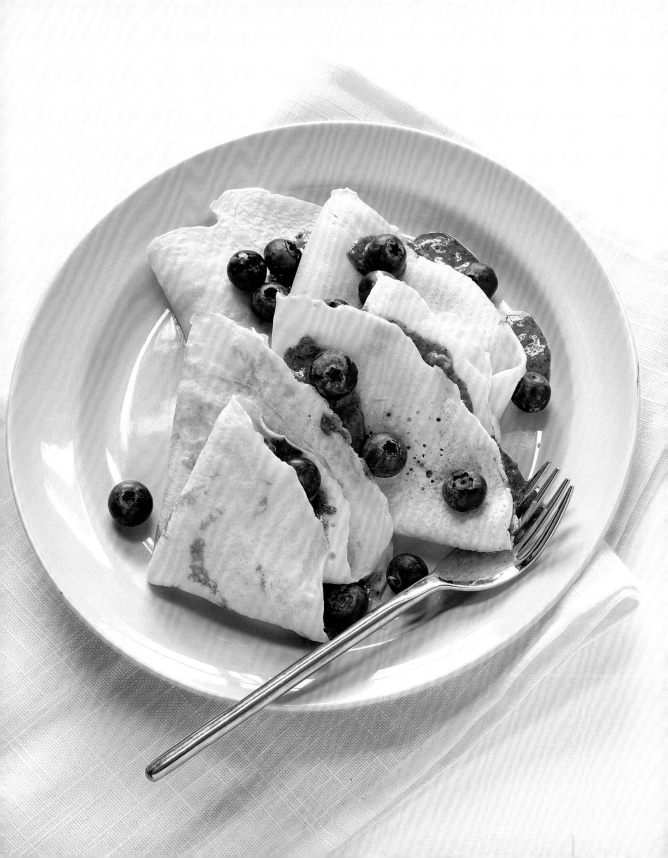

BLUEBERRY PROTEIN CREPES

Ready in 10 minutes
Makes 3 servings

4 egg whites
1 scoop whey protein powder
2 packets Stevia
1 tbsp cinnamon or unsweetened cocoa powder
1 tbsp natural peanut or almond butter
1 cup blueberries

1. Combine the egg whites and protein in a mixing bowl and mix together until smooth.

2. Pour the mixture into a hot nonstick pan. Cook on medium-high for about 2 minutes.

3. Mix Stevia and cinnamon or cocoa powder with almond butter.

4. Fill the crepe's surface with nut butter mixture and blueberries.

5. Fold crepe over so the berries and nut butter are in the center as filling. Cook for 1 to 2 more minutes before serving.

FIT FACT: *Cocoa powder helps to halt the overproduction of cytokines, proteins that cause inflammation.*

Nutrients per serving:

Calories: 130, Total Fats: 4 g,

Saturated Fat: 0.5 g, Trans Fat: 0 g,

Cholesterol: 10 mg, Sodium: 110 mg,

Total Carbohydrates:13 g,

Dietary Fiber: 3 g, Sugars: 7 g,

Protein: 12 g, Iron: 1 mg

ENERGIZING BREAKFAST WRAP

Ready in 15 minutes
Makes 1 serving

¼ cup low-fat granola
6 oz plain low-fat Greek yogurt
½ cup blueberries
4 medium sliced strawberries
1 (7-inch) whole-grain tortilla or wrap

FIT FACT: *Blueberries are high in anthocyanins, a class of antioxidants that is being studied for its effects on weight control and inflammation.*

Mix granola, yogurt and berries, spoon onto wrap or tortilla and roll up, closing the bottom as you go so the filling won't fall out.

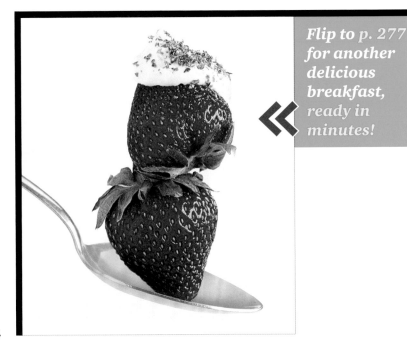

Flip to p. 277 for another delicious breakfast, ready in minutes!

Nutrients per serving:

Calories: 412, Total Fats: 5 g,
Saturated Fat: 1 g, Trans Fat: 0 g,
Cholesterol: 5 mg, Sodium:
446 mg, Total Carbohydrates:
74 g, Dietary Fiber: 6 g, Sugars:
18 g, Protein: 20 g, Iron: 3 mg

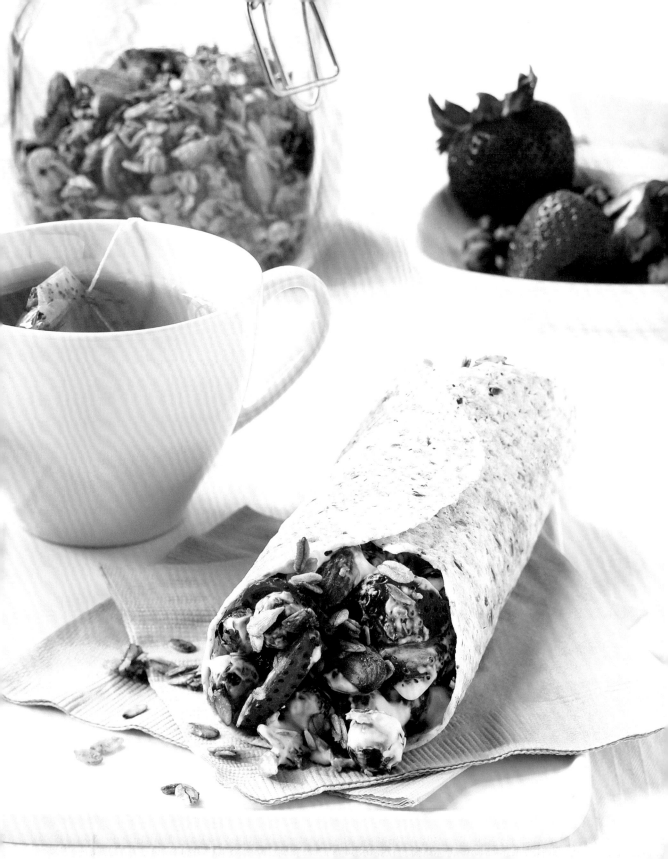

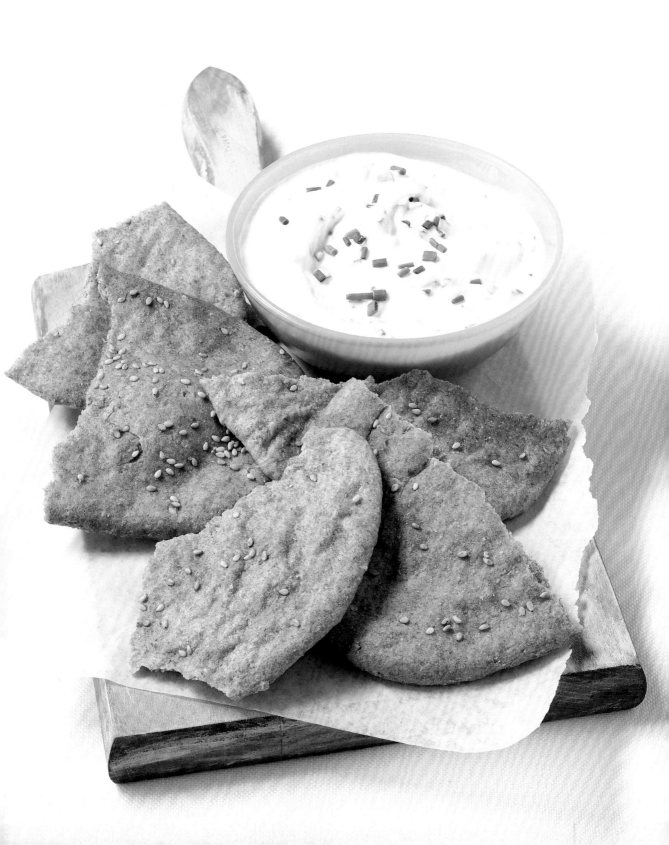

SPELT FLATBREAD WITH YOGURT DIP

Ready in 30 minutes
Makes 8 servings

DOUGH:
⅔ cup lukewarm water
1 tsp dry yeast
1 tsp sea salt
2 Tbsp sesame seeds
1 cup whole-grain spelt flour
½ cup organic fine-wheat spelt flour
4 tbsp extra virgin olive oil

DIP:
1 cup plain nonfat Greek yogurt, to taste
2–4 cloves of pressed garlic
Fresh chopped chives
Salt and pepper, to taste

1. Preheat oven to 375°F. Line a baking sheet with parchment paper.

2. In a large bowl, whisk together dough ingredients thoroughly.

3. Shape dough into four large balls; place on baking sheet. Flatten dough into flat rounds ½- to 1-cm thick. Bake in the oven for about 20 minutes, or until crispy.

4. Meanwhile, mix together dip ingredients in a small bowl. When spelt flats are done, remove and crack in half. Serve chips with yogurt dip.

FIT FACT: *Spelt has a high water solubility, which allows for easy transport of nutrients throughout your body. Like all whole grains, spelt is an excellent source of riboflavin, an energy-revving B-vitamin.*

Dough (8 Servings):
Cal:157, Cals from Fat: 71,
Protein: 3g, Carbs: 17g,
Total Fat: 5g, Sat Fat: 1g,
Trans Fat: 0g, Fiber: 3g,
Sodium: 0g, Cholesterol: 0g,
Sugar: 0g, Iron: 0g

Dip (8 Servings)
Cal: 20, Cals from Fat: 31.5,
Protein: 3g, Carbs: 2g,
Total Fat: 0g, Sat Fat: 0g,
Trans fat: 0g, Fiber: 0.2g,
Sodium: 0g, Cholesterol: 0g,
Sugar: 1.25g, Iron: 0g

KALE CHIPS

Makes 1 serving

2 cups kale, washed and trimmed
1–2 tsp olive oil
Sea salt, to taste

1. Preheat oven to 350°F. Line a cookie sheet with parchment paper.

2. With a knife, remove thick stems from kale and then tear leaves into bite-size pieces.

3. Drizzle kale leaves with oil and massage in, then sprinkle and toss with salt. Roast for 15 to 20 minutes or until crispy. Serve.

FIT TIP: *If you're craving something crunchy and salty, just whip up a batch of these and save yourself the post-potato chip guilt!*

Nutrients per serving:

Calories: 150, Total Fats: 9 g,

Saturated Fat: 1 g, Trans Fat: 0 g,

Cholesterol: 0 mg, Sodium: 0.34 mg,

Total Carbohydrates: 14 g,

Dietary Fiber: 2 g, Sugars: 0 g,

Protein: 4 g, Iron: 0 mg

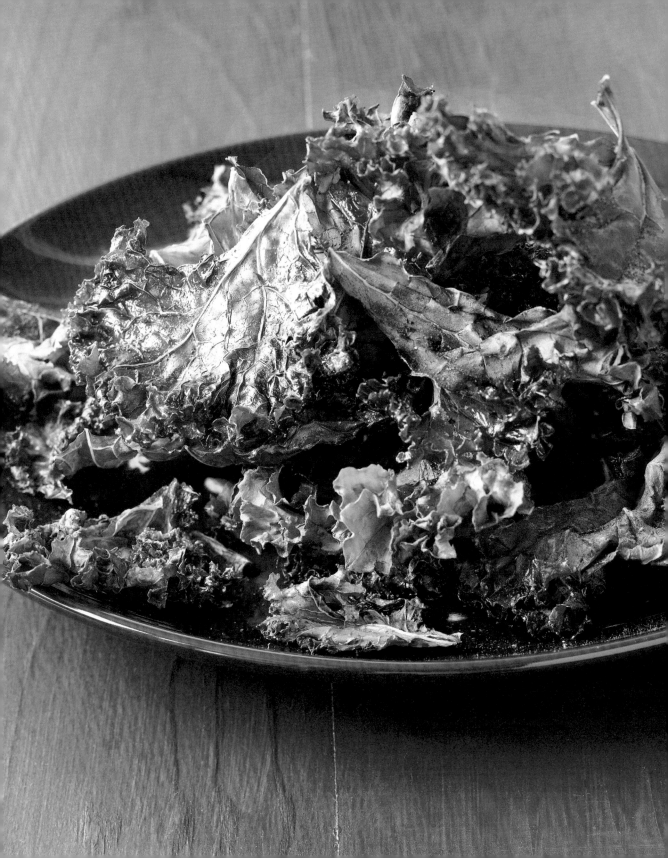

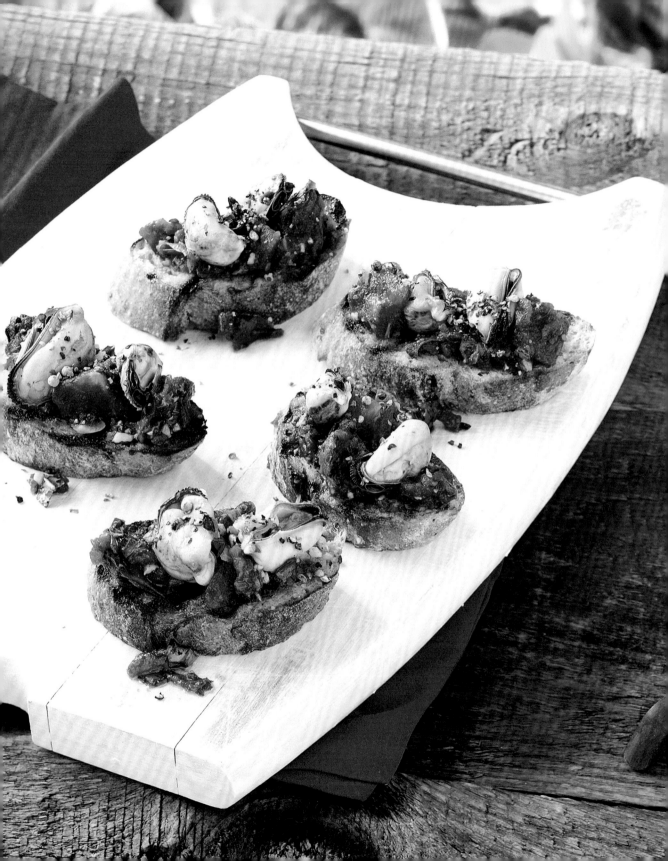

GRILLED MUSSEL BRUSCHETTA

Ready in 1 hour
Makes 4–6 servings

FIT FACT: *Mussels are low in calories and fat, but rich in protein.*

Nutrients per serving:

Calories: 350, Total Fats: 19 g, Saturated Fat: 4 g, Trans Fat: 0 g, Cholesterol: 25 mg, Sodium: 520 mg, Total Carbohydrates: 24 g, Dietary Fiber: 3 g, Sugars: 5 g, Protein: 14 g, Iron: 5 mg

HERB-TOMATO TOPPING:

1 (14.5-oz) can organic fire-roasted diced tomatoes, drained
⅓ cup chopped fresh basil leaves
1 tbsp chopped garlic
1 tbsp chopped oregano leaves
1 tbsp balsamic vinegar
4 tbsp extra virgin olive oil
1 tsp fresh lemon juice
Sea salt and freshly ground black pepper, to taste

MUSSELS:

1 lb small fresh mussels, cleaned and de-bearded
2 tbsp olive oil
1 tbsp unsalted light butter (optional)
3 cloves garlic, minced
1 shallot bulb, minced
⅓ cup white wine

8 thick slices crusty whole-grain bread

1. Mix together herb-tomato topping ingredients in a bowl. Set bowl aside.

2. Set grill on medium-high heat. Make sure all mussels are closed. Tap open ones lightly on a cutting board to close them. If they do not close, discard them.

3. Place a roasting pan on the grill. Add olive oil and butter to pan to melt. Add garlic and shallot and cook, covered, for 2 minutes. Add wine.

4. Add mussels and stir. Grill, covered, for 8 to 10 minutes or until mussels open. Do not overcook.

5. Prepare bruschetta: Brush 1 tsp olive oil on each slice of bread (both sides) and place on grill to toast for 1 to 2 minutes per side. Remove from grill.

6. Shell the mussels.

7. Spoon herb-tomato topping onto bread slices. Top each slice with about 2 mussels, depending on size. Serve.

EASY & ELEGANT TUNA BITES

Ready in 30 minutes
Makes 1 serving

1 (3-oz) can water-packed flaked tuna
1 egg white
⅓ cup shredded carrot
⅓ cup chopped onion
⅓ cup diced tomatoes
⅓ cup chopped leek
Sea salt and freshly ground black pepper, to taste
Cooking spray
4 cucumber slices
Thin slices of melon and cucumber for garnish

1. Preheat oven to 350°F.

2. In a bowl, mix together tuna, egg white, carrots, onions, tomatoes, leeks and seasoning.

3. Shape mixture into 4 balls and press each ball onto an oiled baking sheet. Bake for 20 minutes.

4. Serve on top of cucumber slices. Garnish with thin slices of melon and cucumber, as shown.

FIT FACT: *Eating tuna or salmon just twice a week may boost your omega-3 levels just as effectively as popping a fish oil supplement every day.*

Nutrients per serving:

Calories: 100, Total Fats: 0.5 g,

Saturated Fat: 0 g, Trans Fat: 0 g,

Cholesterol: 15 mg, Sodium: 70 mg,

Total Carbohydrates: 9 g,

Dietary Fiber: 2 g, Sugars: 4 g,

Protein: 14 g, Iron: 1 mg

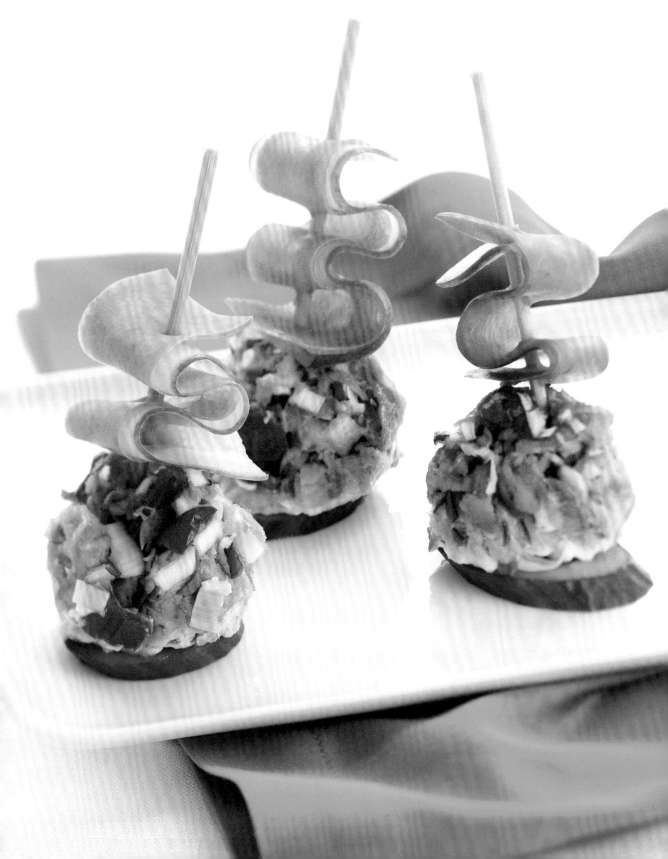

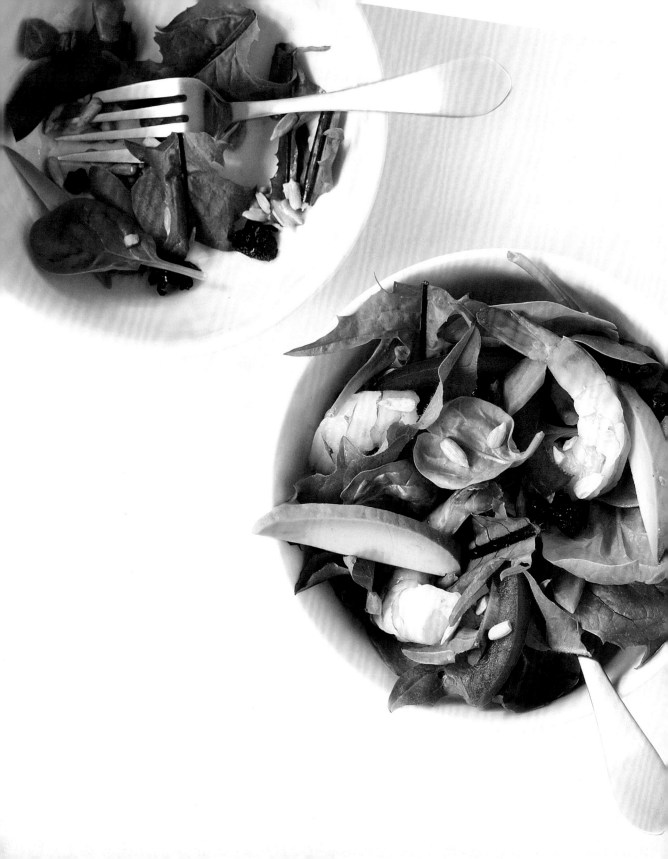

ANTI-STRESS SHRIMP SALAD

Ready in 15 minutes
Makes 2 servings

6 cups spinach
1 cup dandelion greens, washed and trimmed
1 whole red bell pepper, sliced
2 medium carrots, peeled and chopped
¼ cup dried cranberries
1 whole avocado, sliced
2 tbsp raw sunflower seeds
8 oz precooked shrimp
4 tbsp light honey Dijon mustard dressing

1. In a large salad bowl, mix together spinach and dandelion greens.

2. Mix in pepper, carrots and dried cranberries.

3. Top with avocado, sunflower seeds and shrimp.

4. Mix in dressing and serve.

FIT FACT: *Dandelion greens deliver iron, which shuttles oxygen to your working muscles.*

Nutrients per serving:

Calories: 540, Total Fats: 25 g,

Saturated Fat: 3 g, Trans Fat: 0 g,

Cholesterol: 239 mg, Sodium: 600 mg,

Total Carbohydrates: 46 g,

Dietary Fiber: 14 g, Sugars: 22 g,

Protein: 37 g, Iron: 7 mg

CHICKEN & FIRE-ROASTED CORN LETTUCE WRAPS

Ready in 45 minutes
Makes 4 servings

2 boneless, skinless chicken breasts
¼ tsp ground cumin
Juice of 1 lemon
Juice of 2 limes
2 ears corn (yellow or white)
2 plum tomatoes
1 sweet yellow onion, sliced into ½-inch rings
1 jalapeño pepper
1 peach, diced
1 avocado, cubed
½ cup fresh cilantro leaves
Sea salt and freshly ground black pepper, to taste
1 head Bibb lettuce,
    leaves separated into lettuce cups

FIT FACT: *Jalapeño peppers contain capsaicin, the spicy chemical that revs up your metabolism.*

1. Place chicken in a mixing bowl. Add cumin, juice from the lemon and half of the lime juice. Mix to coat and let marinate for 15 minutes.

2. Heat an indoor or outdoor grill to medium-high. Coat grates with canola oil. Grill chicken, corn, tomatoes, onion slices and jalapeño for about 15 to 20 minutes.

3. Remove food from grill. Cut corn off the cob; chop vegetables and chicken into cubes. Optional: remove seeds from jalapeño for less heat.

4. In a large bowl, toss chicken with vegetables, peach, avocado, cilantro and remaining lime juice, to coat. Season to taste. Serve in lettuce cups.

Nutrients per serving:

Calories: 238, Total Fats: 8 g,
Saturated Fat: 1 g, Trans Fat: 0 g,
Cholesterol: 45 mg, Sodium: 258 mg,
Total Carbohydrates: 25 g,
Dietary Fiber: 6 g, Sugars:
7 g, Protein: 21 g, Iron: 1 mg

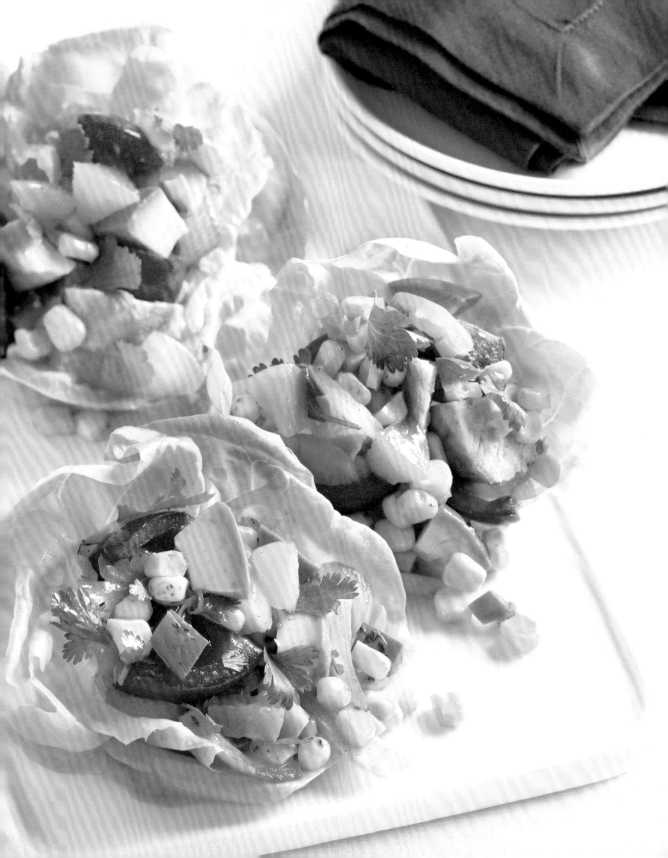

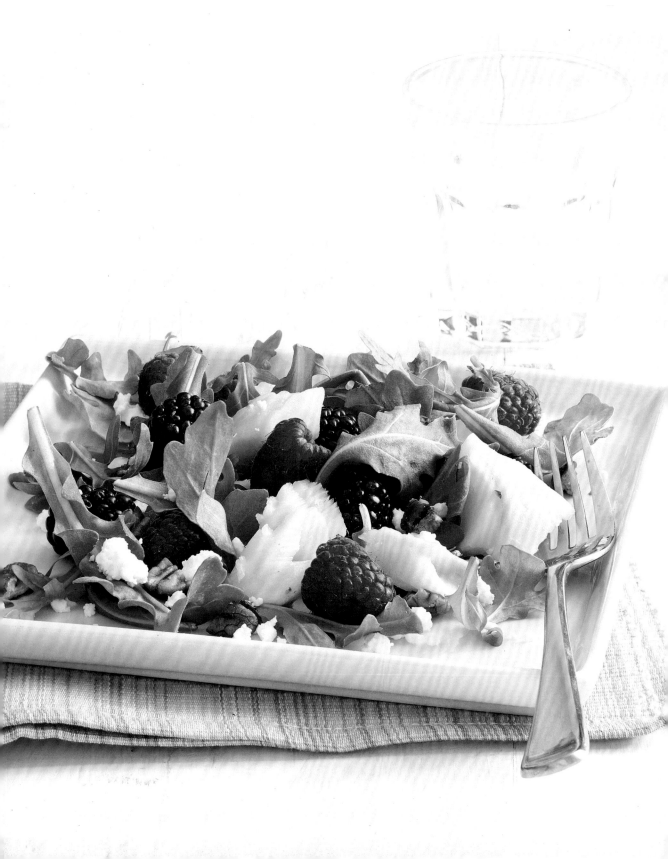

ARUGULA BERRY SALAD WITH STEAMED WHITE FISH

Ready in 15 minutes
Makes 1 serving

4 oz white fish (halibut, haddock, cod or tilapia)
2 cups arugula
1 tbsp balsamic vinegar
½ cup red raspberries
½ cup blackberries
1 tbsp goat cheese
1 tbsp chopped pecans
6 mint leaves; chiffonade leaves by stacking and cutting into
   small ribbons

1. Steam fish until white and flaky, about 5 minutes.

2. In a large mixing bowl, toss arugula with vinegar.

3. Add berries, goat cheese, pecans and chopped mint leaves.
   Transfer salad to a serving plate.

4. Top the salad with fish. Serve.

FIT TIP: *Berries provide anthocyanins, which early studies suggest may help burn fat.*

Nutrients per serving:

Calories: 300, Total Fats: 11 g,

Saturated Fat: 3 g, Trans Fat: 0 g,

Cholesterol: 43 mg, Sodium: 133 mg,

Total Carbohydrates: 21 g,

Dietary Fiber: 9 g, Sugars: 11 g,

Protein: 29 g, Iron: 3 mg

NON-FRIED VEGETABLE QUINOA

Ready in 20 minutes
Makes 1 serving

3 tbsp quinoa
¼ yellow onion, chopped
1 carrot, diced
1 stalk celery, finely chopped, including leaves
1 clove garlic, finely diced
½ red bell pepper, finely diced
1 tsp tamari or low-sodium soy sauce
2 egg whites, beaten
1 whole egg, beaten
1 cup broccoli, chopped small
½ cup water

1. Cook quinoa according to package instructions (should equal about ½ cup cooked).

2. Meanwhile, heat 2 tbsp water in a medium skillet. Steam-sauté onions and carrots for about 5 minutes. Add remaining ingredients except broccoli. Cover and heat for 3 minutes.

3. Add cooked quinoa and broccoli to skillet; add more water to steam. Cover and steam about 3 minutes until the broccoli is bright green. Serve.

Nutrients per serving:

Calories: 350, Total Fats: 8 g,

Saturated Fat: 2 g, Trans Fat: 0 g,

Cholesterol: 212 mg, Sodium: 636 mg,

Total Carbohydrates: 48 g,

Dietary Fiber: 11 g, Sugars: 13 g,

Protein: 25 g, Iron: 6 mg

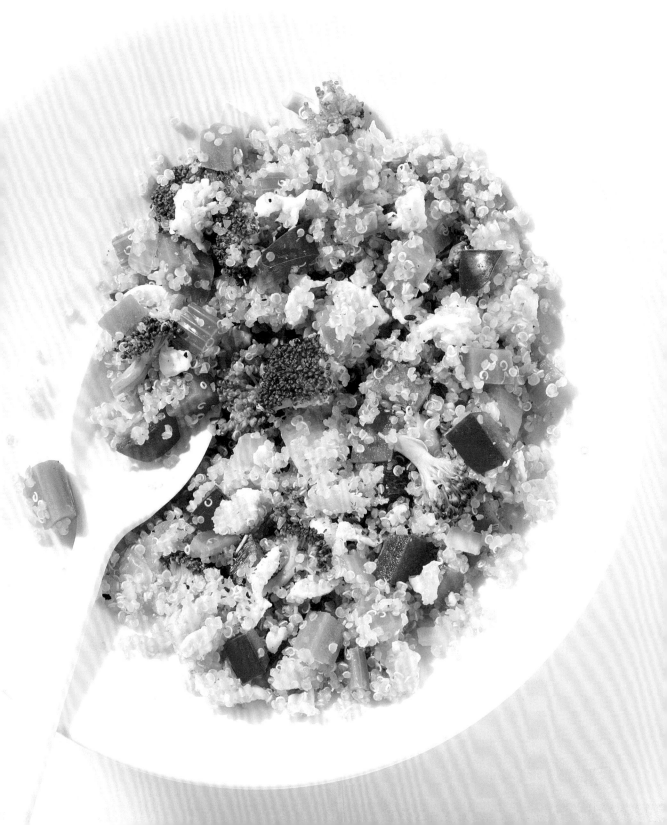

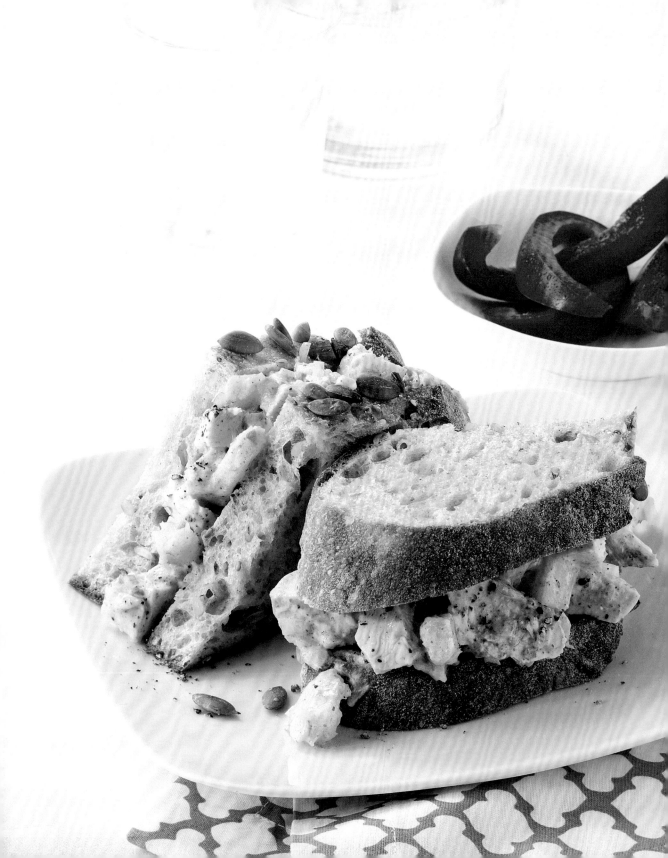

POSTWORKOUT CHICKEN MANGO SALAD SANDWICH

Ready in 15 minutes
Makes 2 servings

6 oz cooked chicken breast
1 small mango
1 small shallot
3 tbsp plain low-fat yogurt
1 tsp curry powder
4 slices whole-grain bread
½ red bell pepper, sliced

1. Chop chicken, mango and shallot into bite-sized pieces. Set aside.

2. In a small mixing bowl, mix together shallot, yogurt and curry powder.

3. Combine yogurt mixture with chicken and mango pieces.

4. Assemble ingredients into two sandwiches. Serve with red bell pepper slices.

FIT FACT: *Mangoes boast vitamins A, B, C and E: an unrivalled stress-fighting nutrient mix among fruits.*

Nutrients per serving:

Calories: 355, Total Fats: 6 g,

Saturated Fat: 2 g, Trans Fat: 0 g,

Cholesterol: 73 mg, Sodium: 530 mg,

Total Carbohydrates: 44 g,

Dietary Fiber: 5 g, Sugars: 21 g,

Protein: 33 g, Iron: 3 mg

SHRIMP & CORN AVOCADO SALAD

Ready in 15 minutes
Makes 4 servings

4 cups romaine lettuce, torn
½ lb cooked shrimp
1 cup corn kernels, cooked and cooled (or use drained canned corn)
1 avocado, cubed

DRESSING:
Juice of 1 lemon (¼ cup)
1 tbsp lemon zest or finely minced peel
2 tbsp balsamic vinegar

GARNISH:
¼ cup chopped cilantro
2 tbsp chopped mint
Freshly ground black pepper, to taste

1. Combine lettuce, shrimp, corn and avocado in a large mixing bowl.

2. Mix in dressing ingredients.

3. Divide among 4 plates.

4. Garnish with chopped cilantro, mint and freshly ground black pepper.

FIT TIP: *When buying shrimp, choose the wild-caught variety for lower mercury and toxin levels.*

Nutrients per serving:

Calories: 185, Total Fats: 9 g,

Saturated Fat: 1 g, Trans Fat: 0 g,

Cholesterol: 111 mg, Sodium: 144 mg,

Total Carbohydrates: 16 g,

Dietary Fiber: 5 g, Sugars: 3 g,

Protein: 15 g, Iron: 3 mg

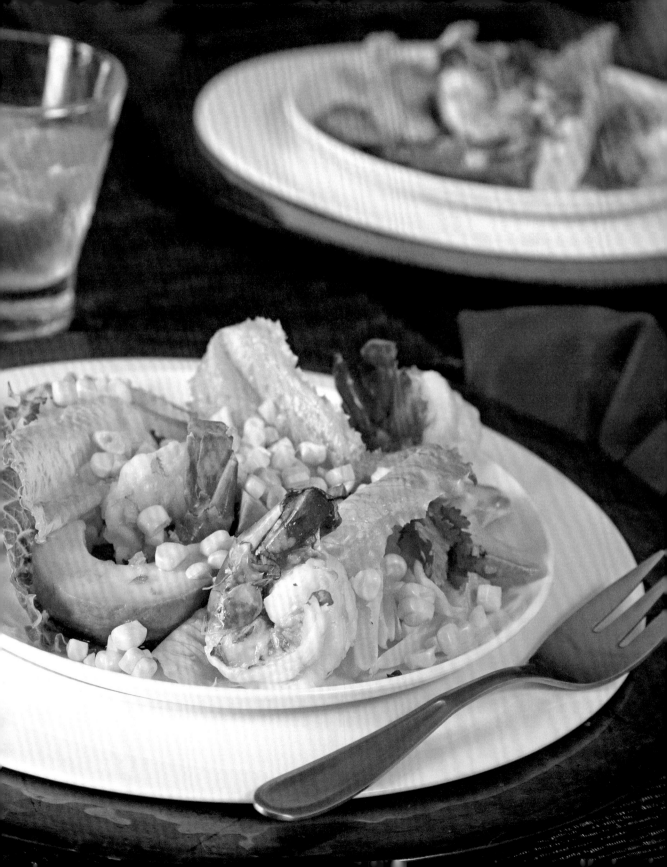

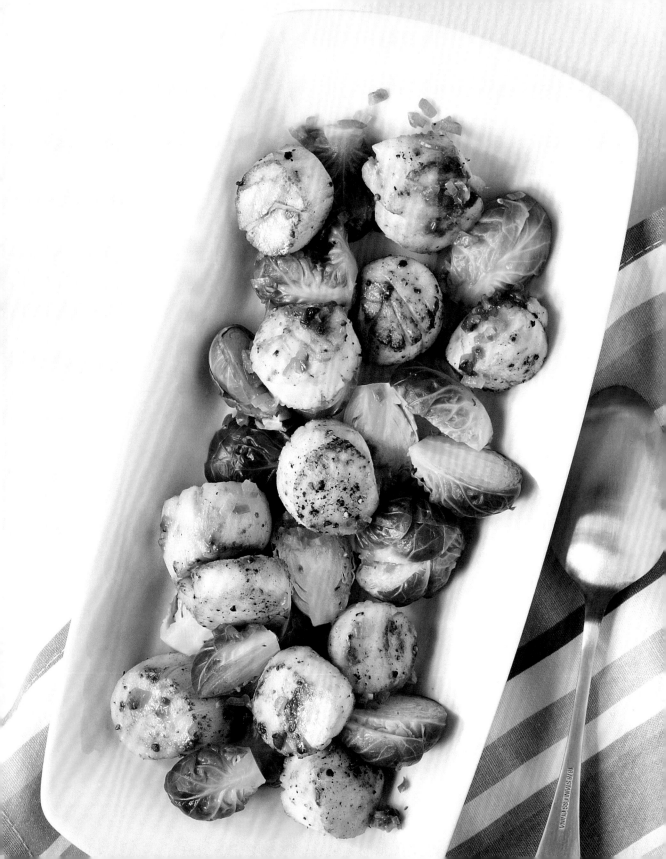

SPEEDY SCALLOPS & BRUSSELS SPROUTS

Ready in 15 minutes
Makes 3 servings

1 lb Brussels sprouts, trimmed and quartered
2 tbsp olive oil
2 tbsp minced shallot
Juice of 1 whole lemon
Freshly ground black pepper, to taste
1 lb sea scallops

1. Place sprouts in a steamer basket and steam in a large saucepan over 3 inches of boiling water until tender, about 10 minutes.

2. In the meantime, whisk oil, shallots, lemon juice and pepper in a bowl.

3. Toss scallops in oil-lemon mix and sprinkle with more pepper, if desired.

4. Place scallops in a skillet preheated to low and brown on both sides, cooking for 10 minutes total.

5. Add the sprouts to the scallop mix and cook for 2 minutes. Serve.

FIT TIP: *Brussels sprouts are loaded with vitamin C, an immunity booster that gets depleted when you're under pressure.*

Nutrients per serving:w

Calories: 210, Total Fats: 8 g,

Saturated Fat: 1 g, Trans Fat: 0 g,

Cholesterol: 35 mg, Sodium: 210 mg,

Total Carbohydrates: 15 g,

Dietary Fiber: 4 g, Sugars: 3 g,

Protein: 23 g, Iron: 2 mg

BEEF TERIYAKI

Ready in 30 minutes
Makes 2 servings

8 oz grass-fed beef, sliced into strips
Juice of 1 lemon
1 tsp olive oil
1 cup water, divided
1 onion, chopped
1 head broccoli, chopped (about 2 cups)
1 bunch baby bok choy, chopped (about 1½ cups)
4 cups kale, chopped
3 tbsp low-sodium soy sauce
1-inch piece ginger, peeled and minced
2 cloves garlic, minced
1 tsp toasted sesame oil
1 lemon, zest and juice
2 tbsp maple syrup
1 tbsp arrowroot powder

1. Place beef strips in a bowl and toss with lemon juice.

2. In a large skillet set on medium heat, brown meat in oil for 5 minutes. Add ½ cup water plus onion, broccoli, bok choy and kale. Cover and reduce heat. Let cook for about 10 minutes.

3. Meanwhile, place remaining ingredients (except arrowroot) plus remaining ½ cup water in a blender and blend to combine. Heat in a small pan.

4. Remove ¼ cup heated sauce and place in a small bowl; whisk in arrowroot with a fork until it dissolves. Stir sauce back into pan and continue stirring until sauce thickens. Pour over beef and vegetables. Serve.

Nutrients per serving:
Calories: 267, Total Fats: 8 g,
Saturated Fat: 2 g, Trans Fat: 0 g,
Cholesterol: 40 mg, Sodium: 613 mg,
Total Carbohydrates: 29 g,
Dietary Fiber: 6 g, Sugars: 12 g,
Protein: 25 g, Iron: 5 mg

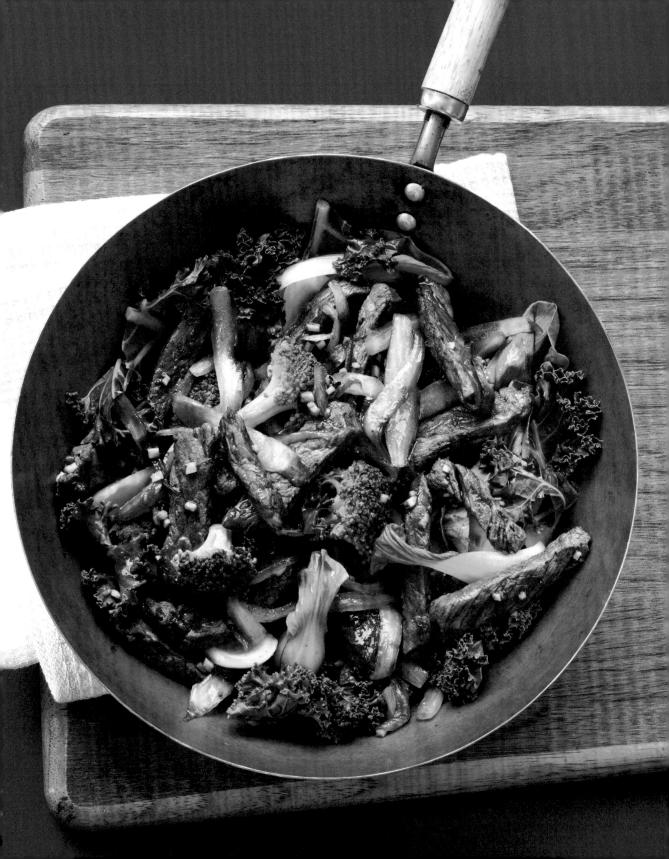

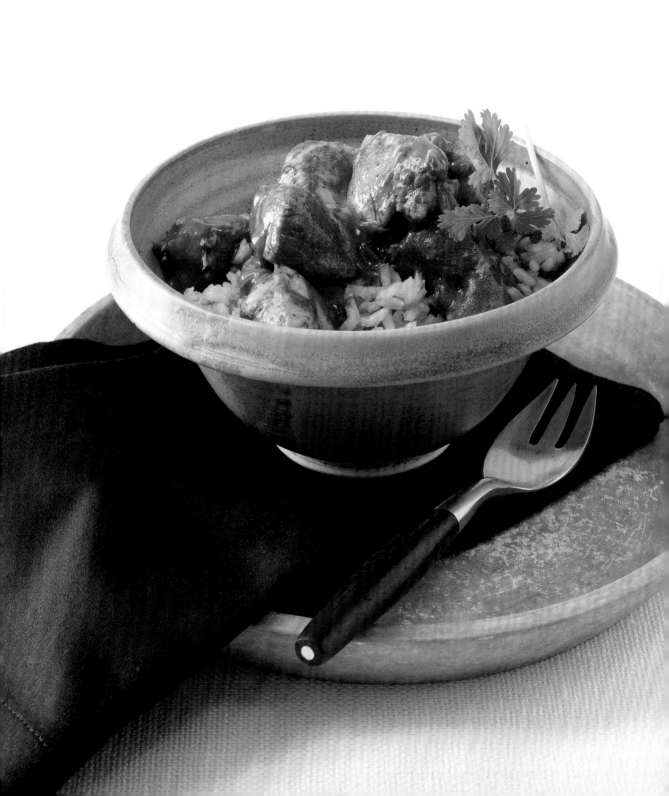

NO-BUTTER CHICKEN

Ready in 20 minutes
Makes 3 servings

12 oz chicken breast, chopped into cubes
Cooking oil
1 small onion, diced
½ tsp minced ginger
1 tsp minced garlic
1 tsp cinnamon
1 tsp turmeric
1 tsp dried coriander
2 tsp paprika
½ tsp cumin
⅛ tsp hot chile pepper
2 tsp low-sodium chicken stock powder
3 tbsp tomato paste
2 tbsp cornstarch
1 cup unsweetened almond milk

1. Sauté chicken in a large skillet coated with cooking oil.

2. Add onion, ginger and garlic, and cook for about 8 minutes, or until fully cooked.

3. Stir in all spices and stock powder. Add tomato paste and fold through.

4. Blend cornstarch with almond milk, then add to pan. Stir continuously until boiled. Add extra milk to thin out sauce, if needed. Cook through and serve.

FIT FACT: *Spices like cinnamon, turmeric and paprika can help reduce high levels of triglycerides (a type of fat in your blood).*

Nutrients per serving:

Calories: 214, Total Fats: 5 g,

Saturated Fat: 0 g, Trans Fat: 0 g,

Cholesterol: 65 mg, Sodium: 160 mg,

Total Carbohydrates: 13 g,

Dietary Fiber: 3 g, Sugars: 5 g,

Protein: 28 g, Iron: 3 mg

CHICKEN SAUTÉED WITH LEEKS & ARUGULA

Ready in 20 minutes
Makes 2 servings

1 (8-oz) chicken breast
2 tsp canola oil
4 tbsp arrowroot powder, divided
3 cups sliced crimini mushrooms,
    stems removed
1 cup thinly sliced leeks, rinsed
    and tough green part discarded
2 cloves garlic, minced
1½ cups thinly sliced shallots
1½ tbsp low-sodium soy sauce
Zest and juice of 1 lemon
6 cups arugula

1. Rinse chicken breast under cool water and pat dry with paper towel. Pound to ½-inch thickness.

2. In a large skillet, heat oil over medium-high heat. Place 2 tbsp of arrowroot on a plate and dredge the chicken to coat thoroughly. Add to skillet and cook until brown, about 2 minutes per side. Transfer to a plate and cover with a lid.

3. Add ¼ cup water to the skillet and use a wooden spoon to remove any brown bits. Add the mushrooms, leeks, garlic and shallots. Sauté for about 5 minutes, adding more water if needed to prevent sticking.

4. Combine remaining arrowroot with soy sauce, lemon juice and zest. Add the mixture to the pan and bring to a boil. Add the chicken back to the pan, reduce heat to simmer and cook another 2 minutes, until the chicken is no longer pink inside. Add the arugula at the end, cover with a lid and steam for 1 more minute. Serve.

Nutrients per serving:
Calories: 421, Total Fats: 9 g,
Saturated Fat: 2 g, Trans Fat: 0 g,
Cholesterol: 87 mg, Sodium: 600 mg,
Total Carbohydrates: 44 g,
Dietary Fiber: 6 g, Sugars:
5 g, Protein: 43 g, Iron: 5 mg

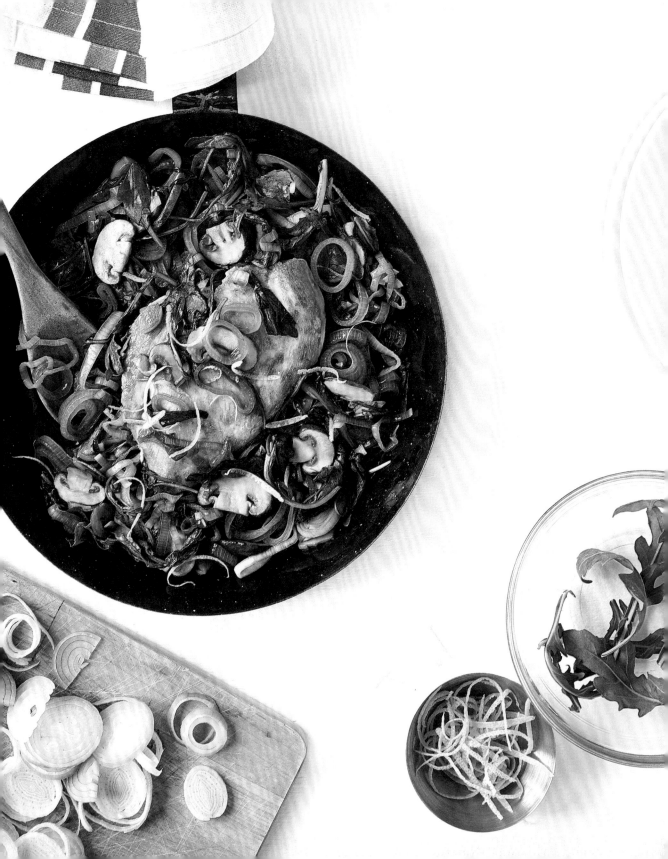

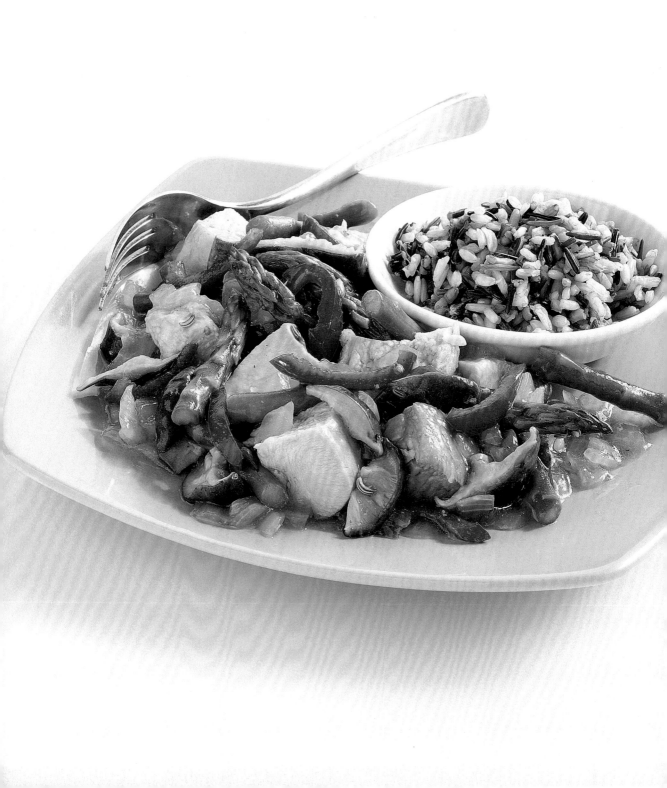

FIVE-SPICE TURKEY

Ready in 30 minutes
Makes 2 servings

2 tbsp olive oil
1 medium onion, chopped
4 cloves garlic, minced
4 cups plus ½ cup water
½-inch piece ginger root, minced
6 whole cloves
1 tsp ground cinnamon
½ tsp star anise
½ tsp fennel seeds
2 (6-oz) boneless skinless turkey breasts, chopped into 2-inch pieces
6 shiitake mushrooms, sliced
1 bunch asparagus, chopped into 1-inch pieces
1 tbsp arrowroot powder

1. Heat oil in a large skillet set on medium-high heat. Sauté onions and garlic for about 3 minutes.

2. Add 4 cups water, ginger, cloves, cinnamon, star anise and fennel seeds. Lower heat and let simmer for 10 minutes to allow broth to infuse with spices.

3. Add turkey pieces, cover with a lid and simmer for about 10 minutes.

4. Mix in mushrooms and asparagus. Cover with a lid to steam, about 3 minutes.

5. Dissolve arrowroot powder into ½ cup water. Add to pot to thicken sauce; add more arrowroot if needed.

6. Serve with brown rice.

Nutrients per serving:
Calories: 358, Total Fats: 9 g,
Saturated Fat: 1 g, Trans Fat: 0 g,
Cholesterol: 59 mg, Sodium: 265 mg,
Total Carbohydrates: 40 g,
Dietary Fiber: 7 g, Sugars:
6 g, Protein: 30 g, Iron: 6 mg

GROUND TURKEY & PASTA PRIMAVERA

Ready in 20 minutes
Makes 1 serving

1 tsp extra virgin olive oil
4 oz extra lean ground turkey
4 oz sliced mushrooms
1 Roma tomato, diced
1 oz baby spinach
1 cup cooked whole wheat pasta
Freshly ground black pepper, to taste
2 tbsp light Italian dressing

1. Heat oil in a skillet set over medium to high heat. Add ground turkey, and cook until brown, about 8 minutes.

2. Add mushrooms and tomato and cook for about 2 minutes. Add spinach and cook for another minute and a half.

3. In a bowl, mix together pasta and ingredients from skillet. Add pepper and dressing. Toss gently to mix.

FIT TIP: *Feel free to use less pasta and more spinach.*

FIT TIP: *Give yourself ample time to digest fiber-rich meals.*

Nutrients per serving:

Calories: 489, Total Fats: 14 g,

Saturated Fat: 2 g, Trans Fat: 0 g,

Cholesterol: 55 mg, Sodium: 550 mg,

Total Carbohydrates: 56 g,

Dietary Fiber: 11 g, Sugars: 3 g,

Protein: 38 g, Iron: 5 mg

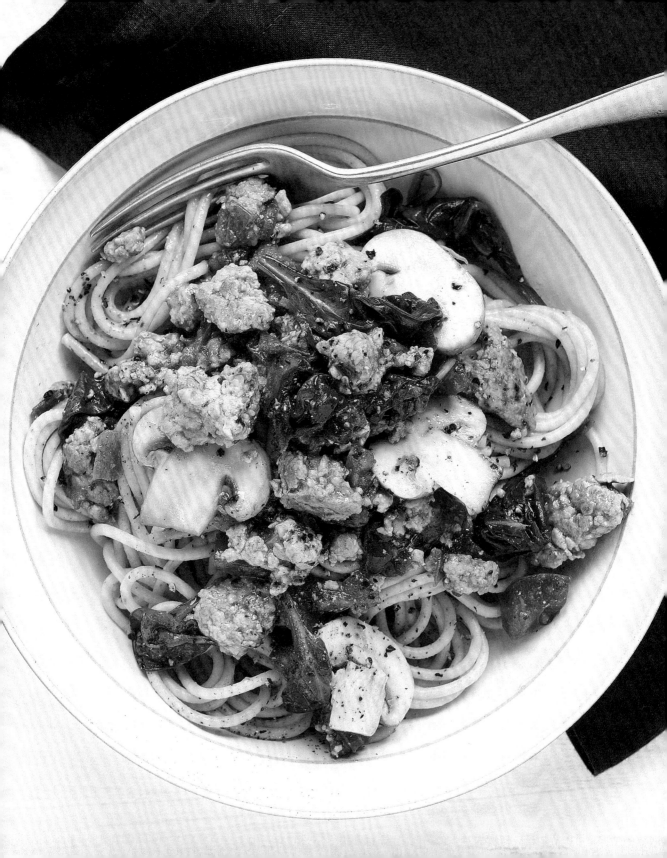

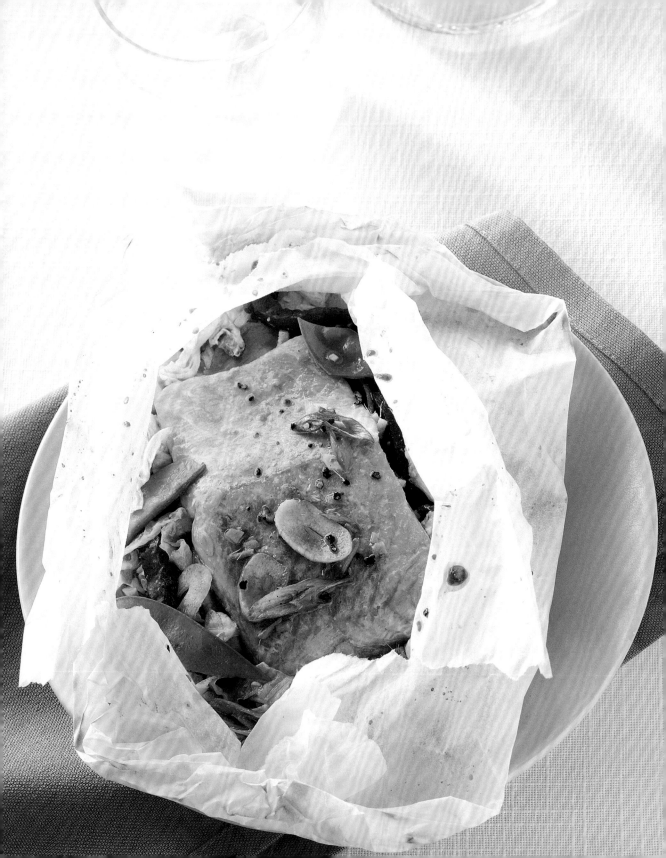

GINGER SALMON IN PARCHMENT PAPER

Ready in 25 minutes
Makes 4 servings

4 cups shredded Napa cabbage
1 red bell pepper, thinly sliced
1 cup snow peas
4 (4-oz) skinless salmon fillets
¼ cup low-sodium soy sauce
1 tbsp minced ginger
2 scallions, chopped
1 clove garlic, sliced
1 tsp sesame oil
¼ tsp freshly ground black pepper

1. Preheat oven to 400°F.

2. Cut 4 large pieces of parchment paper. Fold in half and place equal amounts of vegetables onto each square. Place salmon on top.

3. Whisk remaining ingredients in a bowl and drizzle over fish.

4. Fold in edges to seal and place each closed package onto a large baking sheet. Bake for 20 minutes.

Nutrients per serving:

Calories: 230, Total Fats: 8 g,

Saturated Fat: 2 g, Trans Fat: 0 g,

Cholesterol: 60 mg, Sodium: 660 mg,

Total Carbohydrates: 10 g,

Dietary Fiber: 4 g, Sugars: 5 g,

Protein: 27 g, Iron: 1 mg

PEAR & SAGE-STUFFED PORK CHOPS

Ready in 50 minutes
Makes 4 servings

4 thick, boneless pork chops
¼ cup whole wheat pastry flour
¼ tsp sea salt
⅛ tsp freshly ground black pepper
Olive oil spray
1 Tbsp olive oil
¼ cup yellow onion, chopped
1 stalk celery, minced
1 slice whole wheat bread, cubed
1 pear, cored and diced
1 tsp dried sage
1 tsp fresh rosemary, finely minced

1. Trim away fat and cut a pocket into each chop.

2. Combine flour, salt and pepper on a plate and dredge chops in flour mixture.

3. Sear chops to brown in a skillet sprayed with oil, about 5 minutes on each side. Add some water to pan to deglaze and pull up any brown bits. Remove chops from the pan and set aside.

4. Add oil to pan and sauté onion and celery. Add bread cubes, pear, sage and rosemary. Moisten with 2 tbsp water, or more if needed.

5. Stuff chops with cooked mixture. Place a toothpick in each chop to hold together.

6. Place in a baking dish coated with cooking spray. Pour any residual liquid over chops, cover and bake at 350°F for 30 minutes, until center is no longer pink and internal temperature reaches 145°F. Serve.

Nutrients per serving:
Calories: 231, Total Fats: 8 g,
Saturated Fat: 2 g, Trans Fat:
0 g, Cholesterol: 64 mg, Sodium:
242 mg, Total Carbohydrates:
16 g, Dietary Fiber: 3 g, Sugars:
5 g, Protein: 23 g, Iron: 2 mg

FIT TIP: *For a more festive flavor and about the same amount of calories, replace the pear with a quarter cup of cranberries.*

FIT FACT: *Pork chops used to be on the doctor's hit list, but today they are considered "the other white meat," just as lean as skinless chicken breast. Just look for tenderloin cuts and trim off any visible fat.*

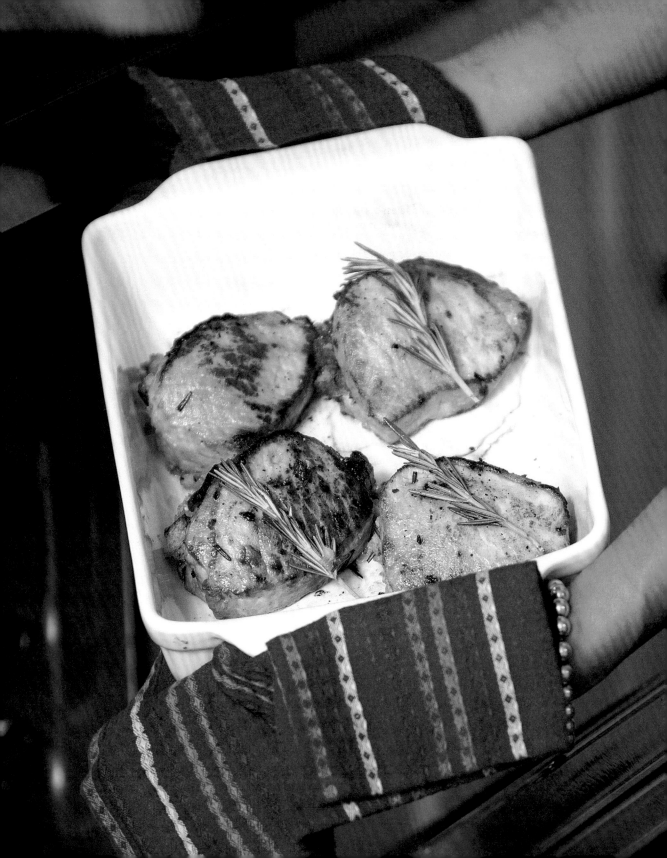

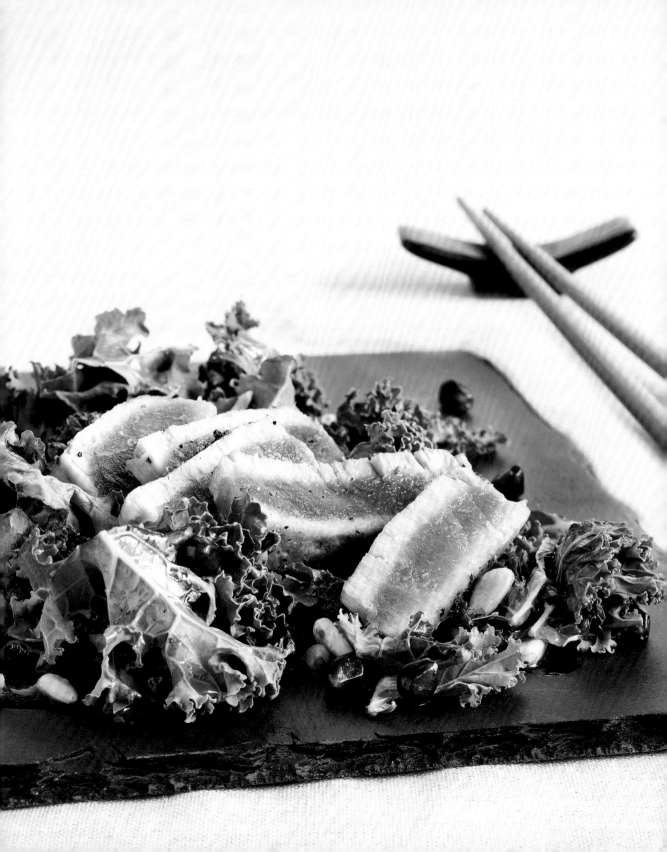

SEARED AHI TUNA ON KALE SALAD

Ready in 25 minutes
Makes 2 servings

3 tbsp pine nuts
1 tbsp olive oil
1–2 tbsp orange juice
Sea salt, to taste
Fresh coarsely ground black pepper, to taste
2 cups stemmed and finely chopped kale
⅓ cup pomegranate seeds
2 (4-oz) ahi tuna steaks (¾" thick)
2 tbsp canola oil

1. Set a cast-iron or other nonstick skillet on medium heat. Add pine nuts and toss until lightly brown. Remove from heat and set aside in a small bowl.

2. In a medium mixing bowl, toss together olive oil, orange juice, sea salt, pepper, kale and pomegranate seeds. Add roasted pine nuts and mix to combine.

3. Season both sides of the tuna steaks with a pinch of sea salt and freshly ground pepper.

4. Heat canola oil in a heavy skillet over high heat. The pan should be as hot as you can get it. Sear tuna on each side for 30 to 45 seconds. Remove from pan and slice into ¼-inch-thick slices; they will be pink inside. Fan out on top of kale salad. Serve.

Nutrients per serving:

Calories: 442, Total Fat: 31 g,
Saturated Fat: 4 g, Trans Fat: 0 g,
Cholesterol: 51 mg, Sodium: 152 mg,
Total Carbohydrates: 15 g,
Dietary Fiber: 2 g, Sugar: 8 g,
Protein: 31 g, Iron: 3 mg

COMFORTING TUNA CASSEROLE

Ready in 30 minutes
Makes 4 servings

1 small sweet potato
6 tbsp Parmesan cheese
1 tbsp canola mayo
1 tsp Dijon mustard
1 tsp garlic powder
1 tsp ground black pepper
1 cup low-fat milk
1 tsp olive oil
½ onion, chopped
1 cup frozen peas
2 cups cooked brown rice
1 (7-oz) can tuna, drained and flaked

1. Preheat oven to 400°F.

2. Pierce sweet potato and heat in a microwave for approximately 5 minutes or until tender. Scoop out the flesh and mash well with a fork. Set aside.

3. In a large mixing bowl, mix together cheese, mayo, mustard, garlic powder, pepper and milk. Add mashed sweet potato and blend well to get a creamy, orange sauce.

4. Heat oil in a medium-large skillet. Sauté onion until soft, about two minutes. Add peas. Add brown rice to reheat. Stir in sweet potato mixture. Add tuna and mix to combine.

5. Place everything in an 8-inch square baking dish and bake for 20 minutes. Serve on a bed of steamed spinach.

Nutrients per serving:
Calories: 330, Total Fats: 6 g,
Saturated Fat: 1 g, Trans Fat: 0 g,
Cholesterol: 18 mg, Sodium: 274 mg,
Total Carbohydrates: 45 g,
Dietary Fiber: 8 g, Sugars: 9 g,
Protein: 25 g, Iron: 3 mg

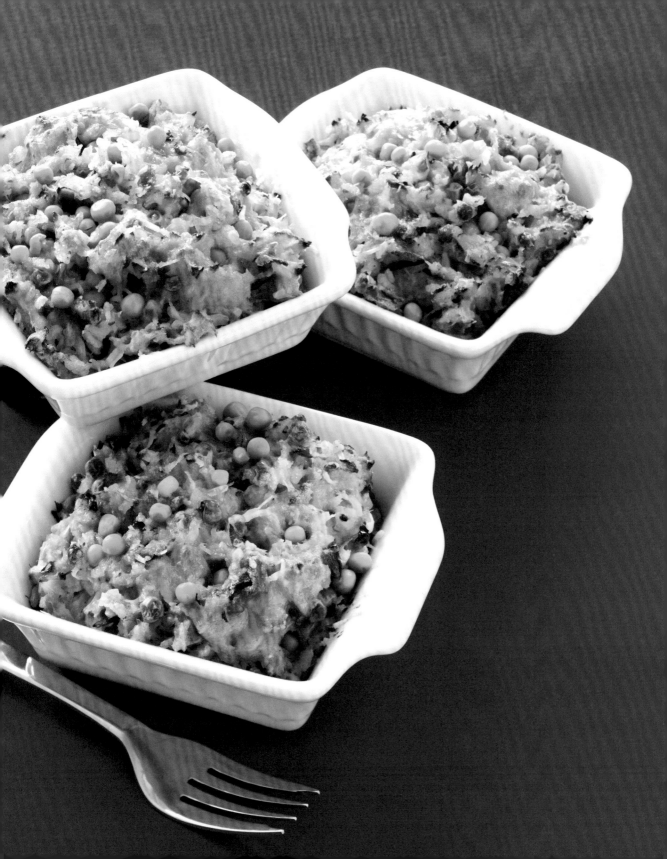

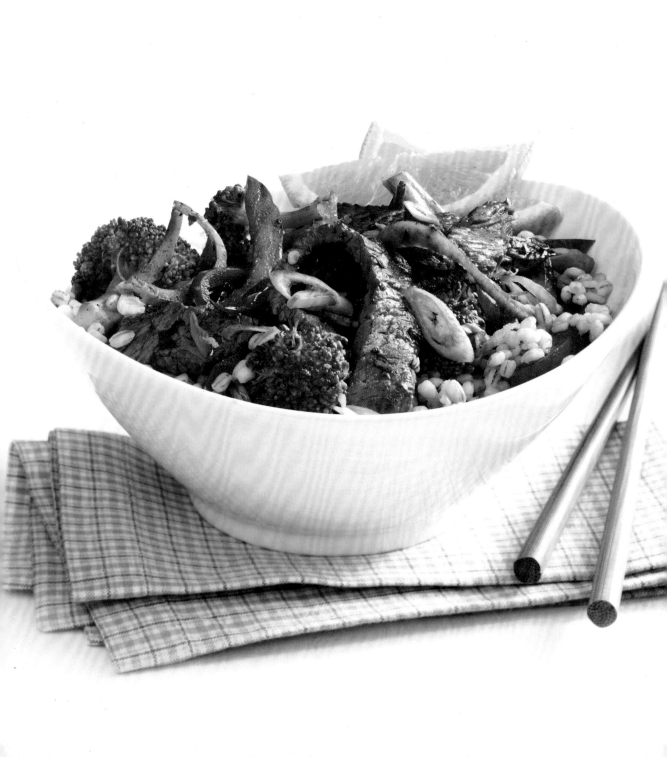

SPICY ORANGE BEEF & BROCCOLI

Ready in 30 minutes
Makes 4 servings

2 oranges
1 tbsp reduced-sodium soy sauce
1 tbsp water
1 tbsp apple juice
1 tsp honey
1 tbsp cornstarch
3 tsp canola oil, divided
½ lb beef sirloin, trimmed of all visible fat
    and sliced into thin slices 1 inch long
4 cloves garlic, minced
1 inch (about 1 tbsp) fresh ginger, minced
1 tbsp dried red pepper flakes (1 tsp for mild spice)
2 heads (about 6 cups) broccoli, chopped
1 red bell pepper, sliced
1 bunch (about ½ cup) chopped scallions with greens

1. Cut ⅛-inch-wide strips of rind from one orange; set aside. Squeeze the juice from both oranges into a small mixing bowl (about ½ cup juice).

2. Whisk in soy sauce, 1 tbsp water, apple juice, honey and cornstarch. Set sauce aside.

3. Heat a large skillet to medium-high and add 1 tsp oil. Add the beef and sauté for 1 minute. Set beef aside on a plate with paper towels to drain excess oil.

4. Add remaining oil to the skillet. Add garlic, ginger, pepper flakes and strips of orange rind and sauté until fragrant, about 30 seconds.

5. Add the broccoli and ⅓ cup water. Cover and steam, about 2 minutes.

6. Add red pepper; sauté for 1 minute.

7. Gradually whisk the orange sauce into the skillet with a fork. Bring to a boil, stirring constantly until sauce has thickened, about 2 minutes.

8. Add the scallions and beef and stir to combine with the sauce. Serve over brown rice or barley.

Nutrients per serving:

Calories: 215, Total Fats: 8 g, Saturated Fat: 2 g, Trans Fat: 0 g, Cholesterol: 46 mg, Sodium: 220 mg, Total Carbohydrates: 17 g, Dietary Fiber: 4 g, Sugars: 8 g, Protein: 21 g, Iron: 3 mg

ITALIAN-STYLE TILAPIA

Ready in 30 minutes
Makes 2 servings

2 large tilapia fillets
14 cherry tomatoes
½ tsp garlic powder
½ tsp dried basil
Sea salt and freshly ground black pepper, to taste
Olive oil spray
½ cup quinoa
2 cups asparagus, ends trimmed

1. Preheat oven to 400°F.

2. Place fillets in an ovenproof glass dish sprayed with olive oil. Place tomatoes on top of the fish.

3. Sprinkle fish with seasonings. Spray olive oil on top and bake for 20 minutes.

4. Meanwhile, steam asparagus and cook quinoa according to package instructions. When fish and tomatoes are done, serve over quinoa with asparagus on the side.

FIT FACT: *Quinoa is a plant-based, gluten-free source of high-quality protein.*

Nutrients per serving:

Calories: 270, Total Fats: 5 g,

Saturated Fat: 1 g, Trans Fat: 0 g,

Cholesterol: 55 mg, Sodium: 410 mg,

Total Carbohydrates: 30 g,

Dietary Fiber: 7 g, Sugars: 5 g,

Protein: 31 g, Iron: 7 mg

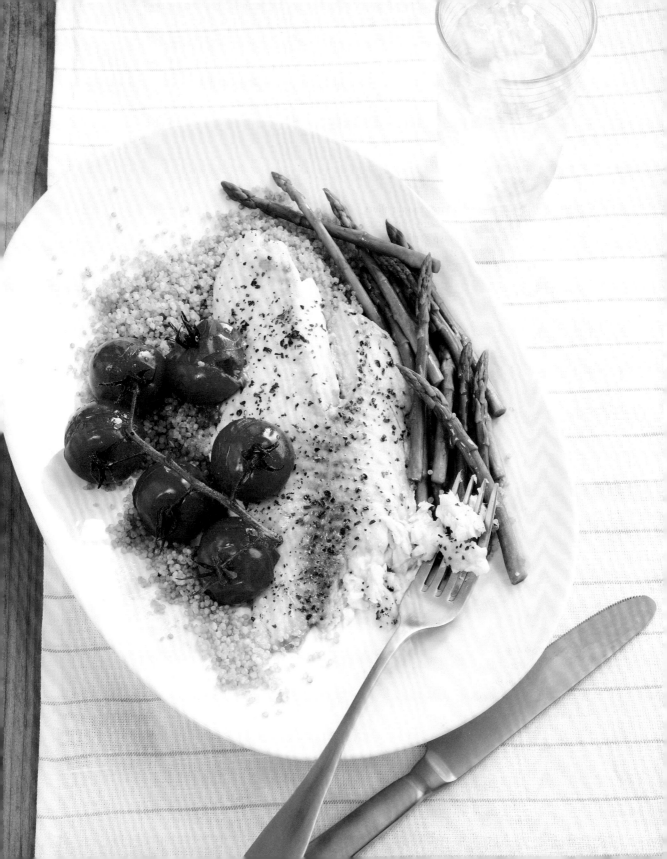

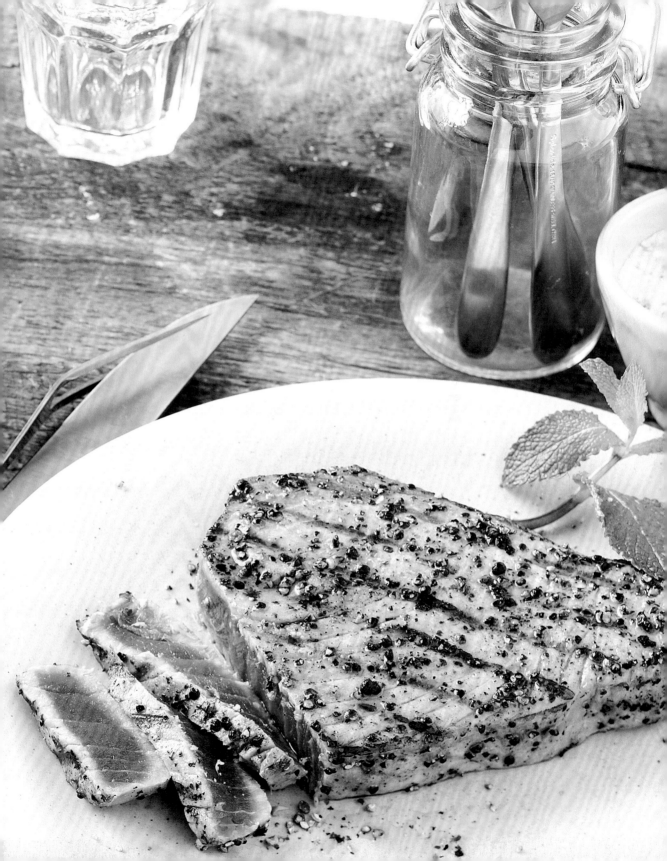

SEARED AHI TUNA WITH CILANTRO-MINT RAITA

Ready in 30 minutes
Makes 4 servings

1½ lb ahi/yellowfin tuna steak(s) (troll or pole-and-line caught are the most sustainable fishing methods)
Coarse sea salt and freshly ground black pepper, to taste
Vegetable oil, as needed
Mint sprigs, lemon and cucumber slices, for garnish

RAITA:
1 cup organic plain low-fat yogurt
½ cup grated English cucumber (unpeeled)
1 clove garlic, minced
2 sprigs fresh mint, leaves only, minced finely
¼ cup finely minced cilantro
½ tsp sea salt
Freshly ground black pepper, to taste

1. Prepare the grill on medium-high heat. Oil a slotted or vented grill pan.

2. In a medium-sized bowl, prepare an ice-water bath. Set aside. Wash and thoroughly dry the tuna. Rub a pinch of salt and a very generous grinding of black pepper on each side (including vertical sides) of the tuna steaks.

3. Prepare the raita by whisking the yogurt until smooth. Add the rest of the ingredients. Stir and chill.

4. Place grill pan on grill and heat on high — make very hot. Sear the tuna on the grill pan on all sides for about 1½ minutes per side.

5. Remove tuna from grill and immediately submerge it in the ice bath for about 1 minute. Remove the fish and thoroughly dry it. Cut the fish diagonally across the grain in slices about ⅓-inch thick, and place on plates.

6. Drizzle with raita, garnish and serve.

Nutrients per serving:

Calories: 230, Total Fats: 3 g, Saturated Fat: 1 g, Trans Fat: 0 g, Cholesterol: 80 mg, Sodium: 350 mg, Total Carbohydrates: 5 g, Dietary Fiber: 0 g, Sugars: 5 g, Protein: 43 g, Iron: 4 mg

GRILLED RASPBERRY SALMON

Ready in 30 to 40 minutes
Makes 6 servings

Vegetable oil as needed
1½ pounds wild-caught salmon fillet
2 tbsp extra virgin olive oil
4 tbsp raspberry vinegar
1 large garlic clove, minced
2 tbsp chopped cilantro
½ tbsp low-sodium tamari or soy sauce
1 tsp minced ginger
1–2 tsp kosher salt
Cilantro sprigs, whole raspberries
    and lemon slices for garnish

1 Preheat grill to medium high. Oil a slotted or vented grill pan. Rinse the salmon and pat dry. Place in a glass or ceramic dish.

3. To make marinade, mix together the next 6 ingredients and pour over salmon. Cover and place in the refrigerator for 15 to 30 minutes.

4. Remove salmon from marinade. Rub the skin side with kosher salt and place on grill pan, skin side down. Spoon some of the marinade over the fish and place on grill.

4. Grill 7 to 10 minutes, or until just barely done. Remove from grill and let fish rest for 1 to 2 minutes to finish cooking. Serve garnished with cilantro sprigs, raspberries and lemon slices.

Nutrients per serving:
Calories: 219, Total Fats: 11 g,
Saturated Fat: 2 g, Trans Fat: 0 g,
Cholesterol: 0 mg, Sodium: 1 mg,
Total Carbohydrates: 3 g,
Dietary Fiber: 0 g, Sugars: 2 g,
Protein: 23 g, Iron: 0 mg

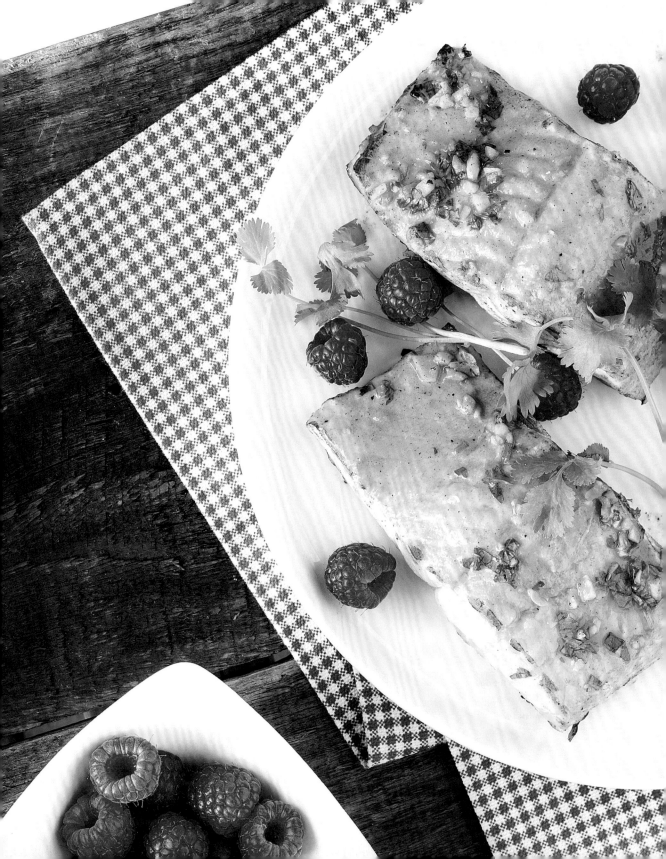

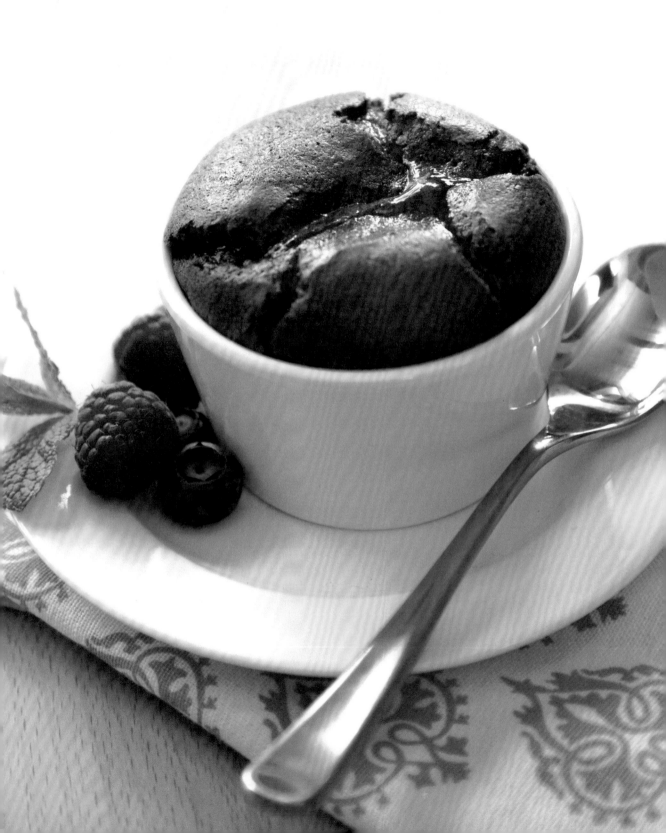

MINI CHOCOLATE SOUFFLÉS

Ready in 30 minutes
Makes 4 servings

Cooking spray
¼ cup unsweetened cocoa
1½ tbsp white wheat flour
½ cup low-fat milk
6 tbsp honey, divided
½ tsp pure vanilla extract
2 large egg whites, cold
⅛ tsp cream of tartar

1. Preheat oven to 350°F. Lightly spray 4 single-serve ramekins.

2. Place cocoa and flour in a saucepan over medium-low heat. Add milk and 3 tbsp honey, and whisk until smooth. Continue stirring until thick, about 2 minutes. Stir in vanilla and set aside to cool.

3. Place egg whites and cream of tartar in a small bowl and beat until soft peaks form. Gradually add remaining honey, continuing to beat at high speed.

4. Fold ¼ cup of the egg whites into the chocolate mixture; gently fold in remaining whites. Divide mixture into prepared ramekins. Bake for 15 minutes, or until puffy and set. Serve immediately.

Nutrients per serving:

Calories: 140, Total Fats: 1 g,

Saturated Fat: 1 g, Trans Fat: 0 g,

Cholesterol: 1 mg, Sodium: 37 mg,

Total Carbohydrates: 33 g,

Dietary Fiber: 2 g, Sugars: 28 g,

Protein: 4 g, Iron: 1 mg

ALMOND BUTTER WHEY COOKIES

Ready in 30 minutes
Makes 12 servings

½ cup oats
1 Tbsp almond butter
1 scoop whey protein powder
1 egg white
2 packets Stevia, or to taste
½ tsp baking powder
⅛ cup carob chips (optional)

1. Preheat oven to 350°F. Line a cookie sheet with parchment paper.

2. Combine all ingredients together in a mixing bowl and mix well with clean hands.

3. Shape the dough into golf-ball-sized balls. Place on the cookie sheet about an inch-and-a-half apart. Bake for about 10 minutes. Serve.

FIT TIP: *Baking with protein powder results in a denser product compared to store-bought cookies and other treats.*

FIT FACT: *Almond butter is packed with monounsaturated fats, shown to suppress hunger.*

Nutrients per serving:
Calories: 30, Total Fats: 1 g,
Saturated Fat: 0 g, Trans Fat: 0 g,
Cholesterol: 5 mg, Sodium: 15 mg,
Total Carbohydrates: 3 g,
Dietary Fiber: 0 g, Sugars:
1 g, Protein: 2 g, Iron: 0 mg

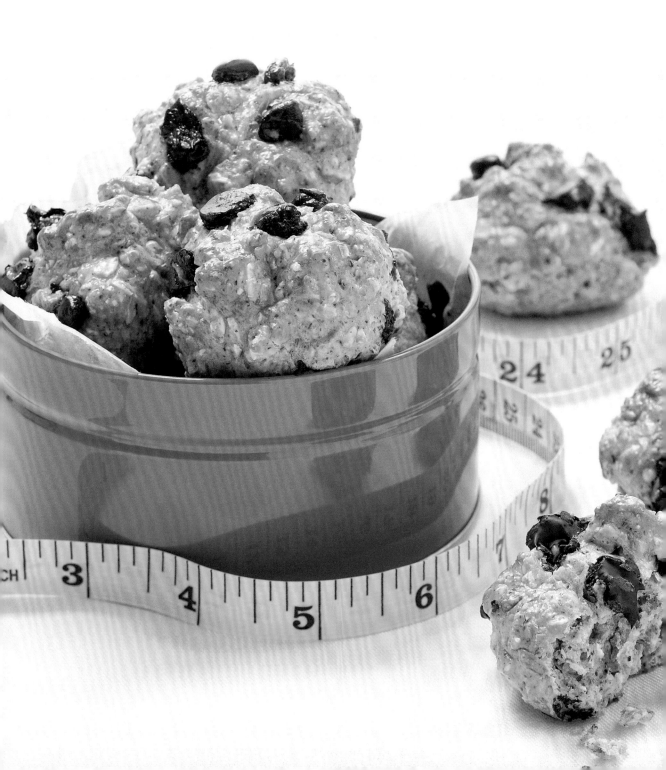

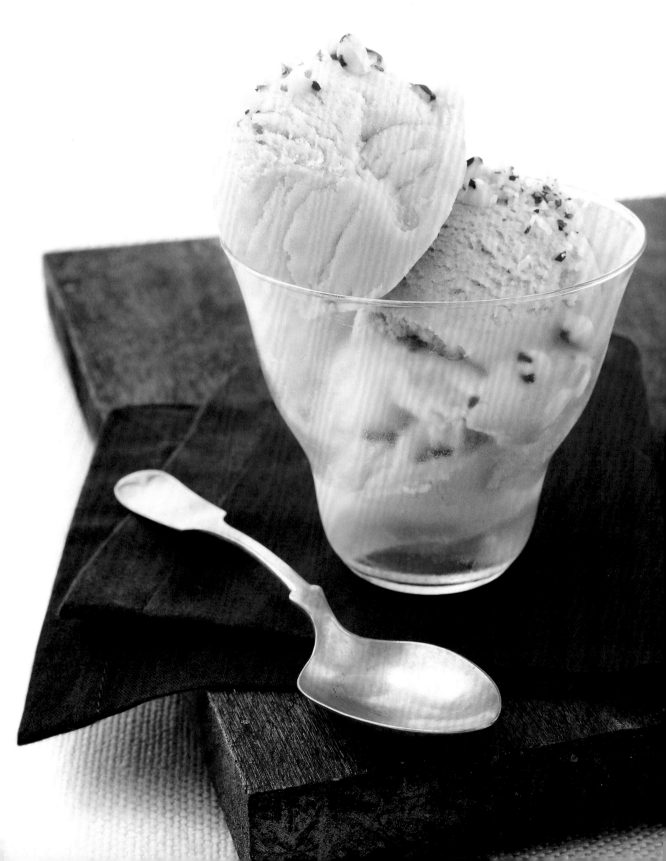

PEPPERMINT PROTEIN ICE CREAM

Ready in 10 minutes
Makes 2 servings

1 cup unsweetened vanilla almond milk
1 scoop vanilla whey protein powder
¼ tsp peppermint extract
¼ cup plain unsweetened 2% Greek yogurt
1 peppermint candy, crushed
½ cup table salt

1. Mix all ingredients, except for peppermint candy and salt, together in a bowl. Or use a blender for quicker results.

2. Pour mixture into a sandwich-sized resealable bag and add the crushed peppermint pieces. Seal the bag. Set aside.

3. Fill a gallon-sized resealable bag halfway with ice. Add ½ cup table salt. Place the small bag into the large bag and seal.

4. Shake the bag vigorously for 5 minutes, until mixture becomes creamy. Remove the bag and rinse off salt. Serve.

FIT FACT: *Unsweetened vanilla almond milk is loaded with the bone-building duo calcium and vitamin D.*

Nutrients per serving:

Calories: 106, Total Fats: 3 g,
Saturated Fat: 1 g, Trans Fat: 0 g,
Cholesterol: 29 mg, Sodium: 142 mg,
Total Carbohydrates: 6 g,
Dietary Fiber: 1 g, Sugars: 4 g,
Protein: 13 g, Iron: 0 mg

CHOCOLATE POWER PUDDING

Ready in 1 hour
Makes 6 servings

4 tbsp chia seeds
12 oz water
1 cup chocolate protein powder
1 cup plain nonfat Greek yogurt
4 tbsp flaxseed meal
2 tsp unsweetened cocoa powder
1 packet Stevia
6 raspberries

1. In a medium-sized bowl, mix chia seeds with water. Let stand for about 20 minutes, stirring frequently, until mixture takes on a gelatin texture.

2. Stir in remaining ingredients, except for raspberries.

3. Chill for about 30 minutes before serving. Garnish with raspberries.

FIT FACT: *The ancient Aztecs considered chia seeds their "running food" because messengers could run around all day on just a handful. Chia seeds are high in hunger-crushing fiber and healthy fats.*

Nutrients per serving:

Calories: 240, Total Fats: 6 g,
Saturated Fat: 0 g, Trans Fat: 0 g,
Cholesterol: 0 mg, Sodium: 540 mg,
Total Carbohydrates: 11 g,
Dietary Fiber: 7 g, Sugars:
2 g, Protein: 37 g, Iron: 1.5 mg

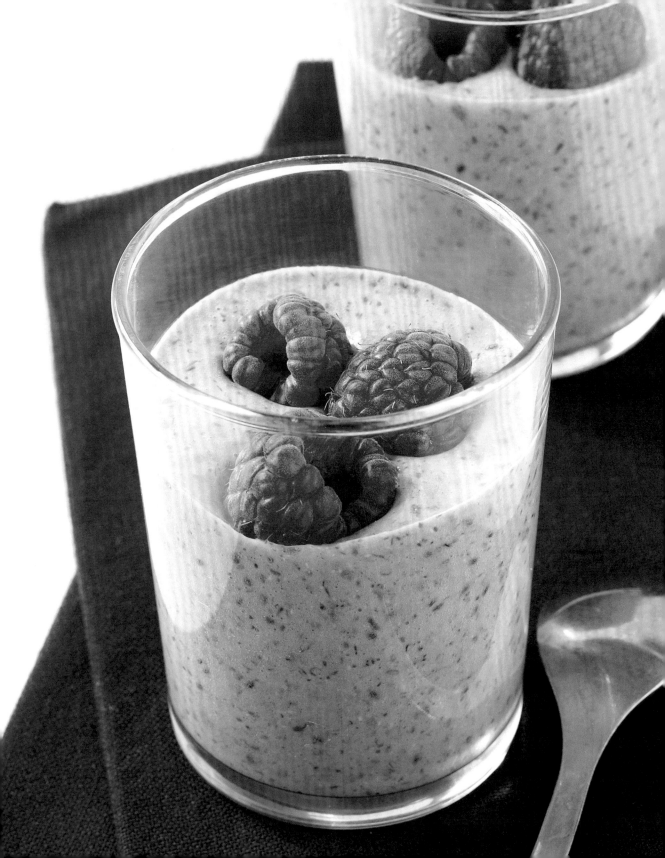

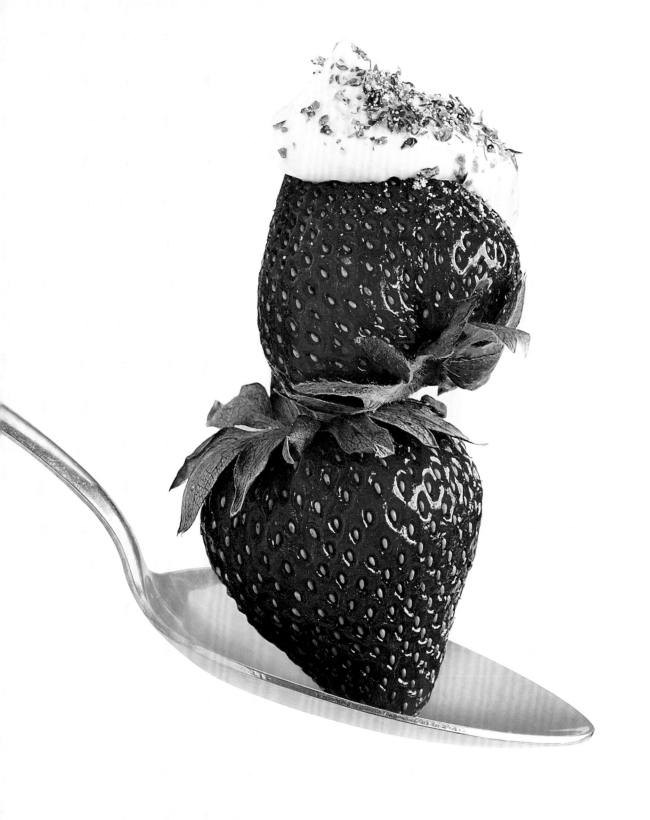

WONDER WOMAN YOGURT PARFAIT

Ready in 10 minutes
Makes 2 servings

1 cup plain low-fat Greek yogurt
½ tsp matcha green tea powder
2 tbsp coconut water
2 tbsp coarsely ground flaxseeds
1 tbsp natural raw honey
2 tbsp natural low-sugar low-fat granola
½ cup sliced fresh strawberries
½ kiwifruit, peeled and sliced

1. In a small bowl, whisk yogurt, green tea powder and coconut water into a smooth paste. Mix in flaxseeds and honey.

2. Spoon granola into a tall glass. Add yogurt to glass.

3. Top with strawberry and kiwi slices. Serve immediately or chill overnight.

Nutrients per serving:

Calories: 213, Total Fats: 5 g,
Saturated Fat: 2 g, Trans Fat: 2 g,
Cholesterol: 0 mg, Sodium: 80 mg,
Total Carbohydrates: 27 g,
Dietary Fiber: 4 g, Sugars:
15 g, Protein: 15 g, Iron: 0.6 mg

Your Vegan and Gluten-Free Options

HOW TO MAKE *THE OXYGEN DIET SOLUTION* WORK FOR YOU!

One of the great things about the diets in this book is that you've got some flexibility when it comes to switching up your meals (For more on this, see the note preceding each meal plan.). You'll also be pleased to know that with a bit of tweaking, all of these diets can be altered to suit a vegan, vegetarian or gluten-free lifestyle. Just follow these guidelines and substitutions.

- When swapping an item, use the same amou... (e.g., replace ½ cup nonfat milk with ½ cup... milk; 2 oz chicken breast with 2 oz tofu at...

- In a pinch, faux vegetarian products ca... cessed items with long lists of artificial...

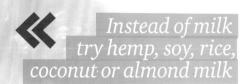

Instead of milk try hemp, soy, rice, coconut or almond milk

VEGAN SUBSTITUTIONS

INGREDIENT	SUBSTITUTE
Cottage cheese	Quinoa with unsweetened almond milk
Eggs (omelette, egg tortilla, egg any style)	Scrambled tofu + 1 tbsp chopped green pepper + 1 tbsp chopped cilantro + 2 tbsp salsa OR 1 slice toasted Ezekiel bread topped with ½ cup black beans + 2 tbsp salsa OR ½ cup cooked oatmeal + ½ cup vegan yogurt + 2 tbsp dried fruit
Meat (chicken, turkey, fish, lamb, steak) and seafood	Tofu, beans, tempeh, textured vegetable protein (TVP), seitan, Sunshine Burgers*, Italian Marinara Beanball Subs (p. 281); for sandwiches, try mixing tempeh or TVP with 1 tsp vegan mayonnaise
Milk	Unsweetened non-dairy beverage, e.g., hemp, soy, rice, coconut or almond milk
Parmesan cheese	Nutritional yeast flakes
Reduced-fat mayonnaise	Reduced-fat vegan mayonnaise
Sirloin burger	Italian Marinara Beanball Subs (p. 281) or another all-natural veggie burger (Try: Sunshine Burgers*)
Subway "Fresh Fit" sandwich	Subway Veggie Delite sub or salad with avocado
Yogurt (Low-fat/nonfat/Greek yogurt)	Any non-dairy yogurt, e.g., Greek-style cultured coconut milk yogurt, soy yogurt, almond yogurt

*This brand of all-natural burgers is organic and vegan. They can also be crumbled or sliced and used as a salad topper.

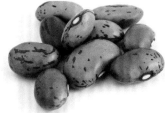

GLUTEN-FREE SUBSTITUTIONS

INGREDIENT	SUBSTITUTE
Bulgur	Quinoa or millet
Cereal (Kashi 7 Whole Grain Puffs)	Gluten-free cereal
Crackers/crispbreads	Gluten-free crackers/crispbreads
Muesli	Gluten-free muesli (Try: Muesli Fusion's Morning Zen)
Oat bran bread	Whole-grain gluten-free bread, brown rice cakes
Oatmeal	Uncontaminated oats, grits, quinoa
Pasta	Rice, corn or quinoa pasta; buckwheat noodles
Soy sauce (low sodium)	Gluten-free tamari
Subway sandwich	Order any of the gluten-free, protein-containing salads and request "double the protein"
Whole-grain slider bun	Gluten-free slider buns; ½ of a regular-sized gluten-free bun (serve open-faced)
Whole-grain toast	Whole-grain gluten-free bread, brown rice cakes
Whole wheat tortilla	Corn tortilla, brown rice tortilla

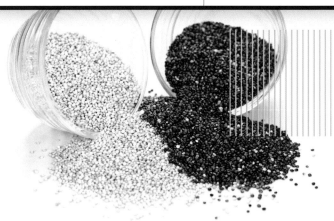

Tosca Reno's daughter Rachel doesn't splurge on treats very often; that's why she likes this clean, vegan version of the classic Italian meatball sub – it's guilt free! The following recipe is from Tosca's *The Eat-Clean Diet Vegetarian Cookbook*, which contains over 150 delicious – and clean – vegan recipes, as well as a wide variety of vegetarian, pescatarian and gluten-free meals.

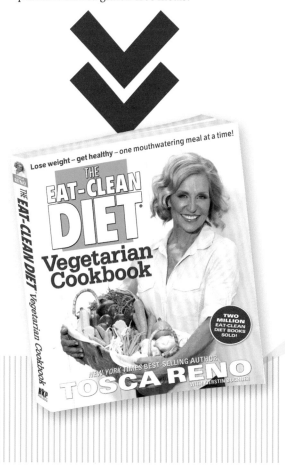

Nutrients per serving (6-inch section of baguette, 4 bean balls, ½ cup marinara):

Calories: 456, Calories from Fat: 94,

Protein: 19 g, Carbs: 77 g, Total Fat: 11 g,

Saturated Fat: 1 g, Trans Fat: 0 g, Fiber: 9 g,

Sodium: 871 mg, Cholesterol: 0 mg

ITALIAN MARINARA BEANBALL SUBS

Ready in 35-40 minutes • Makes 5 servings

BEANBALL INGREDIENTS:

½ yellow or white onion, cut into large chunks

2 cloves of garlic, peeled

½ cup basil leaves, packed

½ cup flat leaf parsley, packed

1 x (15-oz) can organic great northern, white kidney or cannellini beans, drained and rinsed

1 cup cooked red quinoa

2 tbsp Bragg Liquid Aminos

2 tbsp nutritional yeast, plus more to garnish

Pinch red pepper flakes

¼ cup whole wheat dry bread crumbs

¼ cup + 2 tbsp wheat germ

2 tbsp extra-virgin olive oil

¼ tsp each sea salt and freshly ground black pepper

5 x 6-inch sections of whole-grain baguette, sliced in half lengthwise, keeping enough of the bread intact to create a hinge

1½ cups any jarred clean marinara sauce

1. Preheat the oven to 350°F.

2. To a food processor, add onion, garlic, basil and parsley. Pulse chop until smooth. Scrape into a large bowl. Add beans to processor and pulse chop until chunky. Scrape out into bowl. Add remaining Beanball ingredients to bowl and stir to combine thoroughly. Roll 1 beanball to check the consistency. If mixture is too moist to easily hold its shape, add 2 tbsp more bread crumbs and 1 tbsp more wheat germ, and stir to combine. Once the mixture has the right consistency, roll into golf-ball-sized balls and place on a baking sheet lined with parchment. Bake 35 to 40 minutes, until firm to the touch and lightly browned.

3. To assemble subs, pour ½ cup of marinara inside each section of baguette, add 4 beanballs and top with a sprinkle of nutritional yeast, if desired. Serve hot.

Personal data

Keep track of your progress by recording your body measurements each month. The scale doesn't always reveal the truth!

→	DATE	DATE	DATE
WEIGHT			
BODY-FAT PERCENTAGE			

MEASUREMENTS

CHEST			
WAIST			
HIP (at largest point)			
RIGHT THIGH			
LEFT THIGH			
RIGHT ARM - Relaxed:			
- Flexed:			
LEFT ARM - Relaxed:			
- Flexed:			
RIGHT CALF			
LEFT CALF			
FOREARM			

Personal data

→	DATE	DATE	DATE
WEIGHT			
BODY-FAT PERCENTAGE			

MEASUREMENTS

CHEST			
WAIST			
HIP (at largest point)			
RIGHT THIGH			
LEFT THIGH			
RIGHT ARM - Relaxed:			
- Flexed:			
LEFT ARM - Relaxed:			
- Flexed:			
RIGHT CALF			
LEFT CALF			
FOREARM			

Goals

DATE

Setting goals is the key to success. Each goal is a stepping stone toward your ideal self. Give yourself reasonable goals to work toward. Rather than trying to lose 20 lbs in one week, strive for 2 lbs. You can try for 20 lbs over time.

Breaking your long-term goal into attainable short-term goals keeps you aware of your progress, and you are constantly rewarding yourself by completing one step toward a better you!

Weekly Goals

Making positive changes each week will add up.
You'll start seeing results in no time!

By this time next week...

Monthly Goals

Some of your goals will take a little longer. Choose a few monthly goals and stick to the changes you've already made.

By this time next month...

Long-Term Goals

Studies have shown that people who write down their long-term goals are more successful in many aspects of life than those who do not. Do it now!

By this time next year...

Goals

DATE

Setting goals is the key to success. Each goal is a stepping stone toward your ideal self. Give yourself reasonable goals to work toward. Rather than trying to lose 20 lbs in one week, strive for 2 lbs. You can try for 20 lbs over time.

Breaking your long-term goal into attainable short-term goals keeps you aware of your progress, and you are constantly rewarding yourself by completing one step toward a better you!

Weekly Goals

Making positive changes each week will add up.
You'll start seeing results in no time!

By this time next week...

Monthly Goals

Some of your goals will take a little longer. Choose a few
monthly goals and stick to the changes you've already made.

By this time next month...

Long-Term Goals

Studies have shown that people who write down their long-term goals are more successful in many aspects of life than those who do not. Do it now!

By this time next year...

Goals

Setting goals is the key to success. Each goal is a stepping stone toward your ideal self. Give yourself reasonable goals to work toward. Rather than trying to lose 20 lbs in one week, strive for 2 lbs. You can try for 20 lbs over time.

Breaking your long-term goal into attainable short-term goals keeps you aware of your progress, and you are constantly rewarding yourself by completing one step toward a better you!

Weekly Goals

Making positive changes each week will add up.
You'll start seeing results in no time!

By this time next week...

Monthly Goals

Some of your goals will take a little longer. Choose a few monthly goals and stick to the changes you've already made.

By this time next month...

Long-Term Goals

Studies have shown that people who write down their long-term goals are more successful in many aspects of life than those who do not. Do it now!

By this time next year...

Goals

DATE

Setting goals is the key to success. Each goal is a stepping stone toward your ideal self. Give yourself reasonable goals to work toward. Rather than trying to lose 20 lbs in one week, strive for 2 lbs. You can try for 20 lbs over time.

Breaking your long-term goal into attainable short-term goals keeps you aware of your progress, and you are constantly rewarding yourself by completing one step toward a better you!

Weekly Goals

Making positive changes each week will add up.
You'll start seeing results in no time!

By this time next week...

Monthly Goals

Some of your goals will take a little longer. Choose a few monthly goals and stick to the changes you've already made.

By this time next month...

Long-Term Goals

Studies have shown that people who write down their long-term goals are more successful in many aspects of life than those who do not. Do it now!

By this time next year...

Today's training

DATE

EXERCISE	SET 1		SET 2		SET 3		SET 4		SET 5		SET 6		SET 7		SET 8	
	Weight		Weight		Weight		Weight		Weight		Weight		Weight		Weight	
	Reps		Reps		Reps		Reps		Reps		Reps		Reps		Reps	

CARDIO/NOTES:

Today's training

EXERCISE	SET 1	SET 2	SET 3	SET 4	SET 5	SET 6	SET 7	SET 8
	Weight	Weight	Weight	Weight	Weight	Weight	Weight	Weight
	Reps	Reps	Reps	Reps	Reps	Reps	Reps	Reps

CARDIO/NOTES:

MUSCLE GROUPS

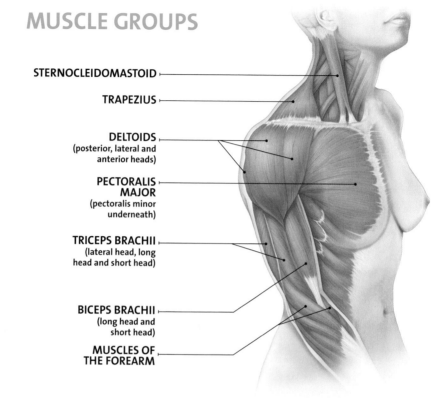

STERNOCLEIDOMASTOID

TRAPEZIUS

DELTOIDS
(posterior, lateral and
anterior heads)

PECTORALIS
MAJOR
(pectoralis minor
underneath)

TRICEPS BRACHII
(lateral head, long
head and short head)

BICEPS BRACHII
(long head and
short head)

MUSCLES OF
THE FOREARM

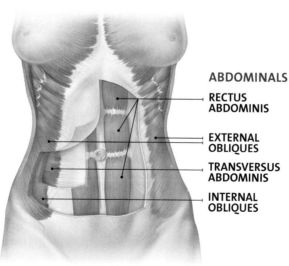

ABDOMINALS

RECTUS
ABDOMINIS

EXTERNAL
OBLIQUES

TRANSVERSUS
ABDOMINIS

INTERNAL
OBLIQUES

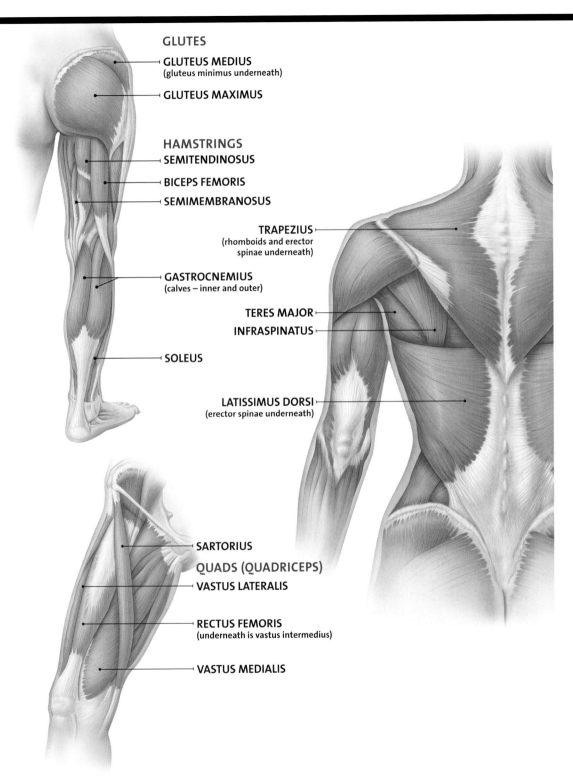

GLUTES

GLUTEUS MEDIUS
(gluteus minimus underneath)

GLUTEUS MAXIMUS

HAMSTRINGS

SEMITENDINOSUS

BICEPS FEMORIS

SEMIMEMBRANOSUS

TRAPEZIUS
(rhomboids and erector
spinae underneath)

GASTROCNEMIUS
(calves – inner and outer)

TERES MAJOR

INFRASPINATUS

SOLEUS

LATISSIMUS DORSI
(erector spinae underneath)

SARTORIUS

QUADS (QUADRICEPS)

VASTUS LATERALIS

RECTUS FEMORIS
(underneath is vastus intermedius)

VASTUS MEDIALIS

Abdominals

The series of muscles located on the lower midsection of the torso. They are used to contract the body forward through a range of six to eight inches, to twist the torso and to hold the torso stable. Together with the lower back muscles the abdominals provide support for posture. The abdominal muscle complex includes the rectus abdominis, transverse abdominis, internal obliques and external obliques.

Aerobic Exercise

Any exercise of relatively low intensity that can be carried out for an extended time and requires oxygen for its energy source.

Amino Acids

Called the "building blocks of life," amino acids are biochemical subunits linked together by chemical bonds to form polypeptide chains. Hundreds of polypeptides, in turn linked together, form a protein molecule.

Anabolic State

Anabolism is a metabolic process whereby smaller units are assembled into larger units. For example, the combining of amino acids into protein strands is a form of anabolism. An anabolic state is one that favors anabolism; for the sake of this book this is a state in which muscle building is possible.

Anaerobic Exercise

Any high-intensity exercise that outstrips the body's aerobic capacity and leads to an oxygen debt. Because of its intensity, anaerobic exercise can be maintained for only short periods of time.

Asymmetric Training

Any exercise that targets only one side of the body at a time. One-arm dumbbell curls are an example.

Barbell

One of the most basic pieces of weight-training equipment. Barbells consist of a long bar, collars, sleeves and associated plates made of steel or iron. They may be either adjustable (allowing the changing of plates) or fixed (the plates are kept in place by welded collars). Barbells weigh between 25 and 45 pounds before adding plates.

Biceps

Flexor muscles located on the upper arm. The biceps is composed of two "heads," and is mainly responsible for bringing the lower arm towards the upper arm across the elbow joint.

Body-Fat Percentage

The percentage of your bodyweight that is made up of fat. On average women have considerably more body fat than men. Here are the commonly accepted body-fat percentage classifications for women, by the American Council on Exercise. Essential fat: 10% to 13%, Athletes: 14% to 20%, Fit: 21% to 24%, Average: 25% to 31%, Obese: 32% or more.

Body Mass Index (BMI)

The measure of an individual's body weight relative to his or her height. A BMI of under 18.5 is considered underweight, a BMI of 18.5 to 25 is considered normal, a BMI of 25 to 30 is considered overweight, and a BMI of over 30 is considered obese. These numbers do not take into account body composition, so a very lean but muscular person may have a higher BMI than a person with a higher body-fat percentage and less muscle.

Buttocks

A term referring to the gluteus maximus, medius and minimus, extensors and abductors of the thigh at the hip joint.

Calorie

Actually a kilocalorie, a calorie is a measure of energy. When you eat, your body converts the caloric energy of food into usable energy or to fat.

Calves

The calves consist of the soleus and gastrocnemius muscles, located on the backs of the lower leg bones. Their function is to plantar flex the ankles.

Carbohydrates

One of three macronutrients that provide energy for the body. Carbohydrates are broken down by the body into glucose, which is then used for energy.

Chest

The large pectoral muscles located on the front of the upper torso, responsible for drawing the arms forward and in toward the center of the body.

Circuit Training

A specialized form of weight training, which combines strength training and aerobic conditioning. Circuit training consists of performing a number of weight-training exercises one after the other, with little rest between sets.

Compound Exercises

Any exercise that works more than one muscle group, over more than one joint. Popular compound movements include: bench presses, squats and bent-over rows. Also referred to as basic exercises.

Cortisol

Catabolic hormone released by the body in response to stress. Cortisol speeds up the rate at which large units are broken down into smaller units (catabolism), and increases fat storage.

Dehydration

Biological state in which the body has insufficient water levels for proper functioning.

Deltoids

The deltoid muscles – anterior, medial and posterior – are located at the shoulder joint. The deltoids are responsible for elevating and rotating the arms.

Diet

A term that refers to a fixed eating pattern. Often used to describe a restrictive food plan followed in order to lose weight.

Dumbbell

Short bar on which weight plates are secured. In most gyms, the weight plates are welded on, and the poundage is written on the dumbbell.

EZ-Curl Bar

Short, S-shaped bar used for such exercises as biceps curls and lying triceps extensions. The bar's unique shape puts less stress on the wrists and forearms than a straight bar.

Fast-Twitch Muscle Fiber

Type of muscle fiber adapted for rapid but short duration contractions.

Fats (Dietary)

One of the three macronutrients that provide energy for the body. Fats have a higher caloric density than protein or carbohydrates. They are necessary for healthy cells, for vitamin and mineral absorption and other bodily functions.

Flexibility

The degree of muscle and connective tissue suppleness at a joint. The greater the flexibility, the greater the range of motion in an individual's limbs and torso.

Forced Reps

An advanced training technique whereby a training partner helps you complete extra reps after the exercised muscles reach the point of fatigue.

Free Weights

Term given to barbells and dumbbells as opposed to weight machines or cables.

Glutes

Another term (with "Buttocks," earlier) referring to the gluteus maximus, medius and minimus, extensors and abductors of the thigh at the hip joint.

Glycogen

Primary fuel source used by exercising muscles. Glycogen is one of the stored forms of carbohydrate.

Hamstrings

The muscle group located on the back of the upper legs, responsible for bringing the lower leg toward the upper leg. The hamstrings are analogous to the biceps in the upper arm.

HIIT

Acronym for high-intensity interval training, a training technique whereby short intense periods of cardiovascular exercise are alternated with easy recovery periods.

Intercostals

Small, finger-like muscles located along the sides of the torso, between the ribs.

Intervals

Periods of more intense exercise alternated with periods of less intense exercise.

Isolation Exercises

Any exercise aimed at working only one muscle and over one joint. In most cases, it's virtually impossible to totally isolate a muscle. Some common examples are: preacher curls, lateral raises, and triceps pressdowns.

Lactic Acid

A byproduct of the anaerobic breakdown of glycogen.

Ligament

Fibrous connective tissue that connects one bone to another over a joint.

Muscle

The series of tissue bellies connected to the skeleton that move and stabilize the body's appendages.

Nutrients

The various minerals, vitamins, proteins, fats, and carbohydrates needed by the body for proper maintenance, health and growth.

Nutrition

The art of combining foods in the right amounts so the human body receives all of its required nutrients.

Obliques

The internal and external obliques work to twist and to laterally flex the torso.

Overtraining

The physiological state whereby the individual's recovery system is taxed beyond its capacity. Among the more common symptoms are muscle loss, lack of motivation, insomnia, an increased heart rate and

Pilates

An exercise system that involves the strength and stabilization of the spine and pelvis, in coordination with strengthening of the muscles and flexibility.

Protein

Nutrient composed of long chains of amino acids. Protein is primarily used in the production of muscle tissue, hormones, and enzymes.

Quadriceps

The quadriceps is the large, four-headed muscle located on the front of the upper legs. The quadriceps primarily work to extend the leg at the knee joint.

Rectus Abdominis

The abdominal muscle we normally think of as the "abs," the rectus abdominis forms the infamous six-pack. Its action is to flex the torso.

Repetition

Normally abbreviated to "rep," this refers to one full movement of a particular exercise.

Resistance

The amount of force being placed on a muscle. In weight training it refers to the amount of weight being lifted.

Set

Term referring to a given number of consecutive reps before resting. Ten nonstop reps would be called one set of 10 reps.

Shocking

Training strategy that involves training the muscle with a new form of exercise. Shocking techniques are used to "kick-start" muscles that have become accustomed to repetitious training routines.

Spinal Erectors

Two long, snake-like muscles located on either side of the spine at the lower to middle back. The spinal erectors work with the abs to maintain posture by extending the joints of the spine.

Split Routines

Any routine for which different muscle groups are worked on separate days rather than working all muscle groups together in one workout.

Stretch Marks

Red or purple lines caused by thinning and loss of elasticity in the skin, normally when there is very fast growth in a specific area. Often caused by pregnancy, weight gain or by breast or hip growth in adolescence.

Strict Form

Training technique which involves performing exercises in a slow, controlled manner, and through a full range of motion, without the aid of a partner or cheating techniques.

Supersets

Advanced training technique whereby sets of two exercises are performed consecutively without rest.

Tendon

A tough cord of connective tissue that connects a muscle to a bone.

Training to Failure

Training on a specific exercise until the muscle simply cannot contract for an additional rep.

Transverse Abdominis

Abdominal muscle that works to stabilize the core, to hold the internal organs in place and to help a woman deliver a baby.

Triceps

Extensor muscles of the upper arm. The triceps are composed of three heads that work in opposition to the biceps – they extend the lower arm and straighten the elbow.

CREDITS

Writers:

Tiffani Bachus, RD (213, 230, 257, 273), Sascha Barboza (226), Meredith Barrett (119-135, 136-141), Monica Bearden, RD (209), Elizabeth Brown, MSC, RD (233, 234, 238, 242, 246, 249, 254, 258, 261), Allison Clark, RD (250), Rachel Crocker (66-69 – plyo workout), Jamie Eason (176-179), Kathleen Engel, NSCA-CPT (70-71, 88-89, 114-115), Kristine Fretwell (245), Diane Hart (162-165), Carina Hultin Dahlmann (221), Nathalie King (253), Kasia Kurek (54-55, 142-143, 166-167, 204-205), Amy Land (12-15, 110-113, 173-175, 180-187, 278-281), Corry Matthews (136-141), Lara McGlashan, CPT (158-161), Alli McKee (48-53), Linda Melone (269), Wendy Morley, (10, 19-21, 26-37, 41-43, 57-60, 73-78, 84-87, 91-93, 98-107, 292-295), Myatt Murphy (32-35), Mindy Parisi (262), Tosca Reno (174-175, 210, 214, 277), Monique Ryan & Helen Vong, 218, 229, 237, 241), Brittany Seki (145-157, 192-201), Gerard Thorne (292-295), Elizabeth Vargas (274), Jennifer Vine (188-189), Allison Young (38-39), Emily Zaler (217, 270)

Cover:

Photographer: Paul Buceta
Model: Lindsay Messina
Hair and Makeup: Valeria Nova
Styling: Rachel Matthews-Burton

Interior:

Biddle, Thomas: 204-205 (Model: Mylene Biddle)

Breeze, Jason: 15 (Model: Olga Svyrydova), 120 (Model: Olga Svyrydova), 124 (Model: Aleisha Hart, Hair & Makeup: Lori Fabrizio), 129 (tip – Model: Lori Harder, Hair & Makeup: Valeria Nova)

Buceta, Paul: 3 (Model: Lindsay Messina), 9 (top: Stacy Kennedy, bottom: Diane Hart, Hair & Makeup: Valeria Nova), 11 (Model: Lindsay Messina, Hair & Makeup: Valeria Nova), 13 (Model: Tosca Reno, Hair & Makeup: Valeria Nova), 14 (Model: Kirsteyn Brown, Hair & Makeup: Valeria Nova), 31 (Model: Lindsay Messina, Hair & Makeup: Valeria Nova, Stlying: Rachel Matthews-Burton), 32-37 (Model: Lindsay Messina, Hair & Makeup: Lori Fabrizio, Styling: Rachel Matthews-Burton), 39 (No Pain

No Gain cover – Model: Amber Elizabeth), 40-41 (Model: Vanessa Pipoli, Hair & Makeup: Valeria Nova), 42 (Model: Julie Bonnett, Hair & Makeup: Valeria Nova, Styling: Nadia Pizzimenti), 49 (Model: Rita Catolino, Hair & Makeup: Valeria Nova & Lori Fabrizio), 50-53 (Model: Lindsay Messina, Hair & Makeup: Lori Fabrizio, Styling: Rachel Matthews-Burton), 56-57 (Model: Lindsay Messina, Hair & Makeup: Valeria Nova, Stlying: Rachel Matthews-Burton), 59 (Model: Tosca Reno, Hair & Makeup: Valeria Nova), 60 (Model: Kirstyn Brown, Hair & Makeup: Valeria Nova), 61 (Model: Francisca Dennis, Hair & Makeup: Valeria Nova), 67-69 (Model: Lindsay Messina, Hair & Makeup: Lori Fabrizio, Styling: Rachel Matthews-Burton), 72-73 (Model: Miryah Scott, Hair & Makeup: Valeria Nova), 78 (Model: April Deweese), 84-87 (Model: Lindsay Messina, Hair & Makeup: Lori Fabrizio, Styling: Rachel Matthews-Burton), 90-91 (Model: Lori Harder, Hair & Makeup: Valeria Nova, Location: Urban Active Polaris, Columbus, OH), 92 (Model: Lindsay Messina, Hair & Makeup: Valeria Nova, Styling: Rachel Matthews-Burton), 93 (Model: Lori Harder, Hair & Makeup: Valeria Nova), 98 (Model: Kirstyn Brown, Hair & Makeup: Valeria Nova), 99 (Model: Lindsay Messina, Hair & Makeup: Valeria Nova, Styling: Rachel Matthews-Burton), 100-107 (Model: Lindsay Messina, Hair & Makeup: Lori Fabrizio, Styling: Rachel

CONTINUED >>

Matthews-Burton), 108-109 (Models – left to right: Rachel Davis, Andrea Brazier, Erica Willick), 110 (treadmill – Model: Kim Dolan Leto), 112-113 (Model: Brittney Layne, Hair & Makeup: Valeria Nova, Styling: Nadia Pizzimenti, Clothing: H&M, Lululemon & Reebok), 118-119 (Models: Rita Catolino & Brooke Stacey, Hair & Makeup: Valeria Nova), 126 (Model: Karen-Lisa Borders, Hair & Makeup: Valeria Nova), 130-131 (Model: Vanessa Pipou, Hair & Makeup: Valeria Nova, Styling: Nadia Pizzimenti), 131 (Model: Jamie Eason, Hair & Makeup: Valeria Nova), 132 (Model: Erin Stern, Hair & Makeup: Lori Fabrizio), 135 (Models: Tosca Reno & Rita Catolino, Hair & Makeup: Valeria Nova), 143 (Model: Lynn Howland – after photo), 144-145 (Model: Sofia Venanzetti, Hair & Makeup: Valeria Nova), 147 (Model: Robert Kennedy), 148-150 (Model: Lindsay Messina, Hair & Makeup: Valeria Nova, Styling: Rachel Matthews-Burton), 151 (Model: Diane Hart, Hair & Makeup: Valeria Nova), 153 (tip – Model: Stacy Rinella, Hair & Makeup: Valeria Nova), 153-154 (Model: Lindsay Messina, Hair & Makeup: Valeria Nova, Styling: Rachel Matthews-Burton), 154 (Model: Alicia Harris, Hair & Makeup: Valeria Nova, Styling: Julia Perry, Clothing: Elisabetta Rogiani), 156 (Model: Melissa Hall, Hair & Makeup: Valeria Nova), 157 (Model: Heather Green, Hair & Makeup: Valeria Nova), 158-161 (Model: Stacey Thompson, Hair & Makeup: Valeria Nova, Styling: Nadia Pizzimenti, Clothing: Nike, Lululemon & Adidas), 163 (Model: Rita Catolino, Hair & Makeup: Valeria Nova), 164 (Models: Tosca Reno & Rita Catolino, Hair & Makeup: Valeria Nova), 175 (top – Model: Tosca Reno), 176-179 (Model: Jamie Eason), 179 (tip – Model: Tosca Reno, Hair & Makeup: Valeria Nova), 183 (Quick Tip – Model: Stacey Thompson; Fit Tip – Model: Lori Harder, Hair & Makeup: Valeria Nova), 185 (tip – Model: Nicole Wilkins, Hair & Makeup: Valeria Nova; Get Technical – Model: Karen-Lisa Borders, Hair & Makeup: Valeria Nova), 187 (Model: Tosca Reno), 195 (Model: Karen-Lisa Borders, Hair & Makeup: Valeria Nova), 202 (Model: Kirstyn Brown), 203 (Model: Rachel Crocker), 206-207 (Model: Brooke Griffen), 239 (Food Styling: Claire Stubbs), 255 (Food Styling: Claire Stubbs), 268

Chou, Peter: 215 (Food Styling: Claire Stubbs, Prop Styling: Madeleine Johari), 216 (Food Styling: Claire Stubbs, Prop Styling: Genevieve Wiseman), 220 (Food Styling: Claire Stubbs, Prop Styling: Genevieve Wiseman), 231 (Food Styling: Claire Stubbs, Prop Styling: Genevieve Wiseman), 271 (Food Styling: Claire Stubbs, Prop Styling: Genevieve Wiseman)

Farr, Ken: 189 (Model: Cindy Flannery – after)

Flannery, Bill: 188 (Model: Cindy Flannery – before)

Grigsby, Allen: 55 (Model: Abby Huot – after)

Hager, Tim: 70-71 (Model: Alison Hager)

James, Gregory: 13 (Models: Dave Bowden, Natalie Amaral, Erin Lutz, Savithri Sastri, Hair & Makeup: Jessica Colley), 14 (Models: Alaina Chapman, Stacy Jarvis, Marta Ustyanich, Ashley Souter), 175 (tip – Model: Ashley Souter), 184

Jordan Samuel Photography: 89 (Model: Denyse Raynor – after)

Lohre, Rick: 167 (Model: Jenna Dunham – after)

Louzon, Liana: 127 (Model: Chady Dunmore, Hair & Makeup: Angela Veel)

Masterfile: 18-19, 20

NatalieMinhPhotography.com: 115 (Model: Mitchie De Leon – after)

Pond, Edward: 182 (Food Styling: Claire Stubbs, Prop Styling: Madeleine Johari), 212 (Food Styling: Claire Stubbs, Prop Stying: Madeleine Johari), 227 (Food Styling: Claire Stubbs, Prop Styling: Madeleine Johari), 243 (Food Styling: Claire Stubbs), 259 (Food Styling: Claire Stubbs)

Pudge, Jodi: 55 (ahi tuna – Food Styling: Terry Schacht, Prop Styling: Madeleine Johari), 89 (eggs), 115 (pasta), 117, 167 (muffins), 198, 208 (Food Styling: Terry Schacht, Prop Styling: Madeleine Johari), 211 (Food Styling: Ashley Denton), 219 (Food Styling: Terry Schacht, Prop Styling: Jay Junnila), 223, 224 (Food Styling: Terry Schacht, Prop Styling: Madeleine Johari), 228 (Food Styling: Terry Schacht, Prop Styling: Jay Junnila), 234, 236 (Food Styling: Terry Schacht, Prop Styling: Jay Junnila), 240 (Food Styling: Terry Schacht, Prop Styling: Jay Junnila), 247 (Food Styling: Terry Schacht, Prop Styling: Madeleine Johari), 248 (Food Styling: Claire Subbs, Prop Styling: Madeleine Johari), 251 (Food Styling: Terry Schacht, Prop Styling: Madeleine Johari), 252 (Food Styling: Adele Hagan, Prop Styling: Genevieve Wiseman), 256 (Food Styling: Marianne Wren, Prop Styling: Catherine Doherty), 260, 264 (Food Styling: Terry Schacht, Prop Styling: Madeleine Johari), 275 (Food Styling: Adele Hagan, Prop Styling: Madeleine Johari)

Ramos, Gideon: 114 (Model: Mitchie De Leon – before)

Raynor, Adam: 88 (Model: Denyse Raynor – before)

Reiff, Robert: 39 (Model: Kelly Smith, after photo), 136 (Model: Katie Uter-Normand, Hair & Makeup: Teri Groves, Styling: Elisabetta Rogiani), 139 (Model: Katie Uter-Normand, Hair & Makeup: Teri Groves, Styling: Elisabetta Rogiani), 141 (Model: Katie Uter-Normand, Hair & Makeup: Teri Groves, Styling: Elisabetta Rogiani), 168-169 (Model: Koya Webb, Hair & Makeup: Nancy Jambazian, Clothing: Elisabetta Rogiani

Ross, Geoffrey: 192, 194

Shutterstock: 21 (Pixelbliss), 30 (artjazz), 38 (spotlight: Africa Studio), 49 (MaxyM), 54 (goggles: Pashin Georgiry), 58 (kubais), 70 (shoes: val lawless), 71 (pizza: marco mayer), 74 (thermometer: Bart_J, pillows: Africa Studio), 75 (Fatseyeva), 76 (photoinnovation), 77 (TFoxFoto), 78 (Tischenko Irina), 88 (carrot: Anna Kucherova), 98 (bottom: Kitch Bain), 110 (woman with headphones: stefanolunardi), 111 (dumbbells: Stas Tolstnev, pilates class: holbox), 112 (woman with towel: Vadym Drobot), 114 (dumbbells: ArtRoms), 121 (walnuts: bioraven, bananas: Anna Kucherova), 122 (Kitch Bain), 123 (Dana Heinemann), 125 (Ikuni), 127 (woman with towel: Yuri Arcurs), 128 (margarita: svry, woman on bicycle: Olga Danylenko), 129 (woman in bed: Ana Blazic Pavlovic), 132 (journal: vetkit), 133 (Natalia Natykach), 137 (Dmitri Mihhailov), 138 (bananas: Maks Narodenko, oats: VikaRayu, cauliflower: geniuscook_com), 140 (asparagus: Sally Scott, chickpeas: Galayko Sergey), 142 (dumbbells: LitDenis), 143 (milkshake: Zadorozhnyi Viktor), 151 (groceries: Monticello), 152 (suitcase: Danny Smythe, cocktail: artjazz), 156 (airplane: MO:SES), 157 (oats: Seregam), 171 (stockshoppe), 181 (water: Tischenko Irina), 184 (Supri Suharjoto), 188 (clock: ronstik), 193 (Jezper), 195 (leaves: Vitaly Korovin), 199 (Ambient Ideas), 200 (hemp: jurgajurga, flax seeds: Africa Studio), 201 (wheat germ: Imageman, fish: kzww), 204 (weight: koya979), 278 (kubais), 279 (Teresa Azevedo), 280 (Elena Elisseeva)

Visnyei, Maya: 17 (Food Stlying: Ashley Denton), 174 (Food Styling: Ashley Denton), 179 (pepper), 180 (Food Styling: Claire Stubbs) , 186 (Food Styling: Claire Stubbs), 196-197 (Food Styling: Claire Stubbs), 205 (shake), 218 (Food Styling: Adele Hagan, Prop Styling: Genevieve Wiseman), 244 (Food StylingL Terry Schacht, Prop Styling: Madeleine Johari), 263 (Food Styling: Ashley Denton, Prop Styling: Jay Junnila), 272 (Food Styling: Terry Schacht, Prop Styling: Madeleine Johari), 276 (Food Styling: Adele Hagan, Prop Styling: Genevieve Wiseman)

Volland, Stewart: 4-5 (Model: Nicole Costa, Hair & Makeup: Nancy Jambazian, Styling: Julia Perry, Clothing: Lululemon), 26 (Model: Natalie Waples, Hair & Makeup: Christine Copeland), 27 (Model: Melissa Cary, Hair & Makeup: Nancy Jambazian, Styling: Julia Perry, Clothing: Elisabetta Rogiani), 30 (Model: Felicia Romero, Hair & Makeup: Nancy Jambazian), 43 (Model: Nicole Costa, Hair & Makeup: Valeria Nova), 66 (Model: Natalie Waples, Hair & Makeup: Christine Copeland), 149 (tip – Model: Kim Dolan Leto, Hair & Makeup: Christine Copeland), 172-173 (Model: Melissa Pittman)

Werner, Tracy: 38 (Model: Kelly Smith, before)